Cancer Crossings

A volume in the series
The Culture and Politics of Health Care Work
Edited by Suzanne Gordon and Sioban Nelson

For a list of books in the series, visit our website
at cornellpress.cornell.edu.

Also by Tim Wendel

Nonfiction

*Summer of '68: The Season That Changed Baseball, and America,
Forever*

*Down to the Last Pitch: How the 1991 Minnesota Twins and
Atlanta Braves Gave Us the Best World Series of All Time*

*High Heat: The Secret History of the Fastball and the Improbable
Search for the Fastest Pitcher of All Time*

Buffalo, Home of the Braves

Far from Home: Latino Baseball Players in America

*The New Face of Baseball: The One-Hundred-Year Rise and
Triumph of Latinos in America's Favorite Sport*

*Going for the Gold: How the U.S Olympic Hockey Team Won at
Lake Placid*

Fiction

Castro's Curveball

Habana Libre

Red Rain

Books for young readers

Night on Manitou Island

My Man Stan

Cancer Crossings

A Brother, His Doctors, and the Quest for a Cure to Childhood Leukemia

Tim Wendel

ILR Press
An imprint of
Cornell University Press

Ithaca and London

First published 2018 by Cornell University Press

Printed in the United States of America

Library of Congress Cataloging-in-Publication Data

Names: Wendel, Tim, author.
Title: Cancer crossings : a brother, his doctors, and the quest for a
    cure to childhood leukemia / Tim Wendel.
Description: Ithaca : ILR Press, an imprint of Cornell University Press,
    2018. | Series: The culture and politics of health care work | Includes
    bibliographical references.
Identifiers: LCCN 2017034806 (print) | LCCN 2017035540 (ebook) |
    ISBN 9781501711046 (pdf) | ISBN 9781501711053 (ret) |
    ISBN 9781501711039 | ISBN 9781501711039 (cloth : alk. paper)
Subjects: LCSH: Wendel, Eric Gordon, 1962–1973. | Wendel, Tim. |
    Leukemia in children—Patients—New York (State)—Olcott—
    Biography. | Lymphoblastic leukemia in children. | Roswell Park
    Cancer Institute.
Classification: LCC RJ416.L4 (ebook) | LCC RJ416.L4 W46 2018
    (print) | DDC 618.92/99419—dc23
LC record available at https://lccn.loc.gov/2017034806

Cornell University Press strives to use environmentally responsible suppliers and materials to the fullest extent possible in the publishing of its books. Such materials include vegetable-based, low-VOC inks and acid-free papers that are recycled, totally chlorine-free, or partly composed of nonwood fibers. For further information, visit our website at cornellpress.cornell.edu.

For my children, Sarah and Chris,
and my wife, Jacqueline,
for their love and support.

For my parents, Jane and Peter,
who persevered with style and grace.

For my brother Eric and the other
courageous people he found
at Roswell Park.

And what you are growing, here, and there, and over there, are little moments, and the little moments make your memories, and the memories make a life that can't be taken away from you by anyone or anything, not other people's fickleness, not even death.

Joshua Ferris, "The Abandonment"

I made myself remember each thing he did, the way he turned his head, his way of saying things. It was as though I knew it wouldn't be for long. He was from another world—he was a blessing too great for me.

Sebastian Faulks, Birdsong

To see the moon so silver going west,
So ladily serene because so dead,
So closely tailed by her consort of stars,
So far above the feverish, shivering
Nightwatchman pressed against the falling glass.

L. E. Sissman, "December 27, 1966"

Foreword

When three-year-old Eric Wendel was diagnosed with acute lymphoblastic leukemia in 1966, doctors gave his parents the grim verdict that he would survive only a year—eighteen months at best.

Despite the persistence of researchers across the nation, medicine had failed to gain a foothold against this deadly and swiftly progressing disease, which had a mortality rate of 96 percent.

Cancer Crossings tells the story of the physician-scientists whose bold new approach to clinical research ultimately turned that statistic on its head.

But there is another side to this story, one that is deeply personal for author Tim Wendel, because Eric Wendel was his younger brother. That perspective adds depth to the book as Wendel weaves together the science behind the evolution of groundbreaking leukemia treatments and his family's struggle to cope with the uncertainty of Eric's future.

Tim Wendel's skill in writing narrative nonfiction makes *Cancer Crossings* a compelling read for laypeople and medical professionals alike. The book serves as both a loving tribute to Eric and a salute to the extraordinary physicians who tried to save him.

Martin Brecher, MD
Former Chief, Hematology/Oncology Division,
Women and Children's Hospital of Buffalo
Chair Emeritus of Pediatrics,
Roswell Park Cancer Institute

Cancer Crossings

1

Sometime after eight in the evening, with bedtime often come and gone, Dad would stand at the bottom of the stairs and sing out, "I'll beat cha." You would have thought it was a secret command from a pirate movie airing on late-night TV or a cowboy cry from *Roy Rogers* or *Rawhide*. No matter, for the younger kids would come running, eager to beat Dad in another race upstairs to bed.

There were maybe a dozen steps to the old farmhouse's open staircase, and night after night my father would take a short lead only to slow down, almost in slow motion, as he approached the top. Sometimes Dad hung on to win, other times he faltered enough in the stretch for everyone to edge him at the wire. Whoever won would shout out, "I beat cha." Soon enough, the thrill of victory blurred into one word—"Ibeecha!"

That became the name of our first bona fide boat, the one that we sailed together on the inland sea named Lake Ontario. No matter that other boat owners in Olcott, New York, dubbed our vessel "The Anthill," due to all the kids swarming on board. We were *Ibeecha*, filled with confidence and expectations as we learned to keep an eye on the far horizon.

We had so many boats over the years: the Penguin dinghy we tried to sail on the Erie Canal; the 24-foot Shark that first bore us

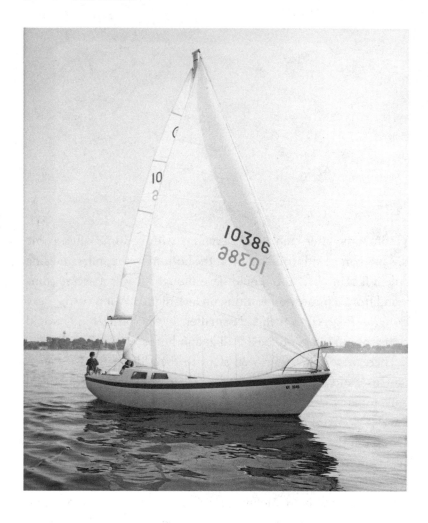

across 40 miles of open water to Toronto; the Cal 27, with its pop-up cabin top, which excelled in light air and sailing downwind, making Dad competitive in the local and Lake Yacht Racing Association races. There were the Cal 3-30 that sported lots of space below deck, including an oven, and the C&C 29, which was better suited for racing than family cruising, much to my mother's regret.

Every man has a sweet tooth, and a sailboat, specifically a gleaming fiberglass job, was my father's. Looking back on it all, my brother Eric shared this affinity for boats more than the rest of us. He and Dad loved to watch crafts of all sizes out on the water, under full sail, looking like so many giant birds in flight.

IN NOVEMBER 1962, only three days before Thanksgiving, my mother gave birth to another boy—Eric Gordon Wendel.

Often parents name their children after family members or dear friends. But Eric was named, in a fashion, after Finnish American architect Eero Saarinen.

"When Mom and I were young, we were fascinated with architecture and the architects of the time," Dad said. "My favorite, and I think Mom's too, was Eero Saarinen. It all began when I learned he and his dad, Eliel, had designed Kleinhans Music Hall in Buffalo. I liked the clean, simple lines of the building that gave it a stately look, and its wood paneling and brick gave it warmth at the same time."

Saarinen also designed the St. Louis Arch, the TWA terminal at JFK Airport, and the Dulles Airport terminal during his short career. With its glass walls, grand open floor, and sweeping, winglike roof, the Dulles terminal stands only 10 miles from my home in northern Virginia, and Saarinen called it "the best thing I've ever done."

Dad said that Saarinen's approach was "to let each building 'tell him what it should be.' He was beyond imposing his ego, his brand, on the building."

In 1961, Saarinen died at the age of fifty-one in Ann Arbor, where he was overseeing a new music building for the University of Michigan. Saarinen died while undergoing an operation for a brain tumor. Eleven years later, his wife, Aline, who was an art critic and television journalist, died of the same condition.

Eero Saarinen's death "hit me pretty hard," Dad said, and he wanted to remember his architectural hero in some way. So when Eric was born, he and Mom briefly considered Eero and Eliel but soon decided those would be difficult names for any kid to deal with. Then they discovered that Eero had a son named Eric. That's what they decided to name my brother.

At first, Eric Gordon Wendel appeared to be like the rest of us. He enjoyed being outside, in motion, always up to something. He laughed as hard as the rest of us at *Quick Draw McGraw* and *Huckleberry Hound* cartoons. Yet his hair was lighter, more reddish in color—a stark contrast to the raven-black mops my brother Chris and I sported. His features were more delicate too. His hazel eyes took in everything, and his lips would draw into a thin smile when something amused him.

In short order, another boy (Bryan) was born, and about five years later a girl (Amy), completing our family of six kids—four boys and two girls. Six kids, if taught the correct procedures, were more than enough to operate a fair-sized sailboat.

On the medical side, our family history couldn't have been better. Both parents were alive and healthy, the grandparents too, and there was no history of allergic tendencies, diabetes, or certainly cancer in our family. So my parents were baffled when Eric could barely get out of bed late in the winter of 1966. He was three years old.

Eric had bruised his right shin during a playdate in the Buffalo suburbs. The blow had deepened and yellowed, lingering on for weeks. Mom took Eric to our family pediatrician, George Muscato, on East Avenue in Lockport, New York. At first, Muscato told my mother that the boy was in fine health, that she was overreacting to some bumps and bruises. But after Mom brought Eric in several more times, the doctor ordered blood work to be done.

Mom had already left Muscato's office when those initial results came in. They indicated a shortage of red blood cells and an alarming platelet count—the telltale signs of leukemia.

Muscato called my father at his office and told him to go home right away and wait for the family station wagon to pull in. Minutes later, when Mom arrived, my parents took Eric straight to Lockport Memorial Hospital. Muscato was waiting for them when they arrived, pacing back and forth in the hallway near the admissions desk.

"I'm sorry," he repeatedly told my mother. "I failed you. I should have listened better."

Another round of blood work confirmed that Eric had acute lymphoblastic leukemia, or ALL. That was a death sentence in the mid-1960s. Under the heading "leukemia" in the *Handbook of Pediatrics* at the time, the diagnosis simply read, "There is no cure for leukemia; treatment is directed at prolonging life and relieving symptoms." The initial prognosis was that Eric would be lucky to live eighteen months.

My brother spent one night at the local hospital, and the medical personnel there didn't know what to do with him. Mom remembered that some of the nurses whispered that he might be contagious. They ordered him to sleep in a crib, with the sides pulled up, tall and tight. They warned him not to climb out—as if they were afraid of him.

The rest of us learned that something was seriously wrong when we came home from school to find our Grandma Bunny making dinner in my mother's kitchen. We knew she didn't think much of that narrow railroad-style kitchen underneath the stairs leading to the second floor. She liked a full room, with plenty of counter space and with the pots and pans and utensils within easy reach.

"Your brother's very sick and your mother's with him at the hospital," she told us after we got off the bus. "I'm making you dinner tonight."

Our house was eerily quiet that evening. Nobody turned on the television after dinner, and there were no Ibeecha races upstairs at bedtime. For the longest time, my younger brother Chris and I tried to drift off to sleep in the bedroom we shared at the time.

"Do you think Eric's going to be OK?" Chris asked.

"I don't know," I replied, trying to sound unafraid. "I don't know."

Early the next morning, April 7, 1966, my parents drove Eric the half hour or so to the Roswell Park Memorial Institute, a few blocks off Main Street in downtown Buffalo.

"We told Eric that we were going to a bigger hospital—one where they could see why he wasn't feeling well," Mom remembered. "We didn't use the word 'cancer.' We never did."

At Roswell Park, Dad signed the papers that detailed how experimental the pending procedures could be. Also, any care at Roswell Park would be free of charge.

"We didn't pay anything," Dad told me years later, "except for gas money."

"No, we paid," Mom added. "We paid with a life."

At Roswell Park, my parents met many of the pediatric doctors. "That morning I was told, 'You're a part of the team,'" Mom said. "That was news to me. I had never been on a team in my life."

2

Why take a long look back, especially to a time when everything in my family seemed to be taken to such extremes? When we seemed to be living well outside ourselves, so far beyond what passed for a normal life? For me, it began with a simple question or two. An interest that opened the door to a past I had largely forgotten or never fully knew.

My daughter, Sarah, was in her first year of medical school, and every other week seemed to bring another examination about another disease that could kill you, a macabre parade of seemingly every malady ever known to man.

"Dad, you had a brother who died, right?" she asked during that period.

Yes, of leukemia, I told her. He died when I was seventeen years old.

"And he was how old?"

He was ten years old. Eric died in 1973.

Thanks to her studies, Sarah knew that kids suffering from leukemia today have a much higher chance of surviving, even enjoying full lives.

"And the doctors, the treatment he received?"

Between the lines, I knew that Sarah was asking if Eric would have been better off at a big-city hospital in New York or Boston.

I told her that my brother had actually been very lucky. He was cared for at Roswell Park in Buffalo, New York, which has long been recognized as one of the best cancer facilities in the country.

"That means your brother was right there, when they were trying to find a cure."

Yes, I suppose he was.

"Don't you see, Dad, they eventually did it. When it comes to leukemia, most kids are now living to be adults."

Eric survived nearly eight years after the original diagnosis—far longer than anybody expected. He was a brave kid, a great brother. But then I had to stop, for I didn't know any specifics in terms of any care and procedures—what my daughter really wanted to discuss. Back then, I wanted to believe that the world was a more equitable, more just place than what played out in what I remember now as the leukemia years. Back then, I was so much in the middle of it all—too afraid to ask too many questions.

After Sarah left that evening, I found an article online in the *New England Journal of Medicine* entitled "Comparison of Intermediate-Dose Methotrexate with Cranial Irradiation for Post-Induction Treatment of Acute Lymphocytic Leukemia in Children." One of its authors was Lucius Sinks, who my mother reminded me was the director of pediatrics when Eric was at Roswell Park. Soon I came across another article, this one from St. Jude Children's Research Hospital in Memphis, for which Donald Pinkel was one of the authors. Pinkel had founded the Department of Pediatrics at Roswell Park in 1956 and was a member of the first multi-institutional group for the study of cancer, the Acute Leukemia Group B.

Sarah had been right. When my brother was diagnosed in the mid-1960s, less than 15 percent of children with the disease survived. Today, that statistic has risen to nearly 90 percent. A wealth of research papers, clinical trials, and scientific journals detailed this amazing turnabout, and many were written by the same doctors—Sinks, Frei, Pinkel, and Holland.

Thanks to forty years of writing for newspapers and magazines and then doing my own books, I've learned how to talk to people and, more important, to listen to what they have to say. If anything, I'm willing to become captivated by "the mad ones," as Jack Kerouac once wrote, "the ones who are mad to live, mad to talk, mad to be saved, desirous of everything at the same time."

In the story of childhood leukemia, a small group of doctors in such locales as Memphis, Boston, Houston, Washington, and Buffalo were known as the mad ones, the ones who dared to take on this shape-shifter of a disease and somehow carry the day. In working my way through the reports and articles, I realized that my brother may have lived only a short while, but he had fallen in with a resilient and determined group of doctors and nurses. As a sportswriter, I've written about many memorable teams: the 1980 Olympic hockey squad at Lake Placid, the 1968 Detroit Tigers, and the St. Louis Cardinals. The list goes on and on.

"You're doing it again," a good friend said. "Investigating a group of underdogs and how they came together. How they overcame great odds."

So where were the leukemia doctors now? How many of these medical pioneers were still working or even alive? What did they think of their efforts years after such procedures and studies had turned the medical world upside down? And what were the points and places where the struggle against childhood leukemia and my family's own story came together?

My daughter's simple question led to so many more. Her interest had taken something from far back in my past and brought it right to the forefront. Over the years, specific remembrances of my brother—the way he smiled, the orderly way he dressed—had faded away. As time had passed, I went weeks, even months, without thinking of my brother. He stayed far in the background until a moment, a simple question, brought him back to the present day again.

Usually when that happened I would briefly reflect on the good times, perhaps when we were all together on the boat, far from shore on Lake Ontario. And then I would let it go. This time, however, I began to think long and hard about those years. How we used to sail across miles of open water in the summer months or skate on the back pond past the railroad tracks when it froze in the winter. How playing softball on a makeshift diamond near the fruit orchards that stretched along Route 18 near Olcott or listening to distant radio stations from Toronto, Detroit, and Chicago reassured me somehow. With those times in mind, I began the search for my brother's doctors.

As with anything, some of it falls into line and the rest becomes much more elusive. Within weeks of Sarah's visit, I returned home to western New York to talk with Dr. Jerry Yates, who had been at the forefront of the early intensive treatments of acute leukemia. We met at the Towne restaurant in downtown Buffalo, only a few blocks from the old *Courier-Express* building, where I had begun my newspaper career.

"Some determined people were involved in this effort," Yates told me. "Unfortunately, we're all getting on in years."

Yates told me about his boss and longtime friend, Dr. James Holland, who at the age of ninety still worked several days a week at Mount Sinai Hospital in New York. Telephone conversations proved to be the best way to speak with Holland.

"After 4:15 in the afternoon until 4:45," Holland said, "that's when I can be found. Call when you can."

Early on I asked Holland why he was still working several days a week, still making the rounds at an elite hospital. A pause followed my attempt at chitchat.

"You have to remember something," Holland finally replied. "Time is always of the essence in any of this. Why am I still going to work in the hospital? Because if I can get a few more years, I sincerely believe I can help find a cure for other cancers. It's always a race, you see."

Beginning in the 1960s and into the 1970s, Holland and Yates spearheaded many crucial advances in leukemia research. That said, they usually worked with adult patients. I needed to find those who were on the fifth floor at Roswell Park, where kids like my brother were treated.

Barbara Hall, one of the first nurses I spoke with, told me about Dr. Donald Pinkel. How he had been Roswell Park's first director of pediatrics before health issues forced him to leave his native western New York and move to western Tennessee, where he founded St. Jude Children's Research Hospital in Memphis. Pinkel now lived in central California, and we began to chat on the phone as well as correspond by email and regular mail.

Still, Pinkel wasn't at Roswell Park when Eric was first enrolled in the rigorous anticancer program there. He had already moved on to Memphis and had begun the uphill fight to build St. Jude. The director of pediatrics during this period in Buffalo was Dr. Lucius Sinks. And when I first started to ask around, nobody knew where he now lived. It took me several months to find out that Sinks lived in Charlottesville, Virginia, only a two-hour drive from my home in suburban Washington. Arguably, the person I needed to talk with the most was almost in my backyard.

I began driving to Charlottesville to meet with Sinks every other month or so. Some friends teased me that Mitch Albom had

Tuesdays with Morrie, while I had "Lunches with Lucius." Sinks and I always got together at the Boar's Head Inn, four miles from downtown Charlottesville. Early on, he didn't know what to make of me or this search for a brother's legacy. I may have met him on one of our family visits to Roswell Park decades before, but neither of us was ever certain. In fact, I wasn't sure of much in those initial conversations at the Boar's Head. The medical terminology, and trying to establish a time line for all that Eric had gone through, was often overwhelming. Yet Sinks was patient with me, and slowly we began to tease things out.

Everyone I spoke with during this search was generous and understanding. Perhaps they realized, as Holland had said, that time was of the essence. That nearly all the medical professionals involved in the campaign to turn the tide against childhood leukemia were in their eighties and nineties now. Certainly a myriad of medical reports, clinical trials, and newspaper stories about this amazing struggle were now part of the public record and will remain forever so. But if I wanted to talk directly with the mad ones who took on and eventually beat ALL, I needed to hurry.

3

To stabilize Eric's condition, the doctors at Roswell Park Memorial Institute first turned to a recognized combination of the old and new—vincristine and prednisone.

Vincristine comes from the periwinkle plant and has a centuries-old reputation in folklore for healing. An alkaloid, bitter in taste, it is an organic substance found in a host of plants in such diverse parts of the world as Canada and the West Indies. These plants sport leafy green leaves and purple flowers. Scientists at Eli Lilly and Company in Indianapolis discovered that vincristine lowers the white blood cell count, and a variation was first used in cancer clinical trials in the early 1960s. When Lilly balked at making it available to a wider audience due to steep production costs, appeals by the National Cancer Institute and hospitals such as Roswell Park put it in play for doctors to fully use. Vincristine was usually given by intravenous injection, and the side effects included hair loss and nausea.

In comparison, prednisone is a synthetic compound that suppresses the immune system and helps relieve inflammation. Unlike anabolic steroids, used by bodybuilders and other athletes, it is a corticosteroid and is effective in treating arthritis, lupus, and difficulties in breathing, as well as childhood leukemia. Prednisone prevents inflammation by sidetracking white blood cells, keeping them from traveling to areas of infection. As a result, long-term use can be devastating to anyone's immune system. Taken in pill form, the possible side effects include increased appetite, which can be beneficial for cancer patients, and swelling, especially in the face, which can be embarrassing for a young kid riding the bus to elementary school. In fact, about the only time Eric ever complained about his situation was after kids on the bus made fun of him.

Vincristine and prednisone work well together. Unfortunately, the effectiveness of the combination against the cancer is short term—lasting only weeks or days before the cancer again gains the upper hand. Although Eric was in no acute distress, the records from this period show, everyone agreed that other measures needed to be taken in a hurry. He was soon enrolled in a clinical trial or protocol, which can be defined as a research project using human volunteers. Eric joined Study No. 6601 at Roswell Park and was given the number 117406. That would remain his patient marker for his seven years at Roswell Park.

Patients in Study No. 6601, about thirty children between the ages of three and thirteen, were scheduled to be shifted over to a regimen of methotrexate or amethopterin given via IV. In the early 1960s, methotrexate was used in combination with three other drugs, including vincristine and prednisone, in a program that was known by the acronym VAMP (vincristine, amethopterin or methotrexate, 6-mercaptopurine [6-MP], and prednisone). In a best-case scenario, this treatment could slow the dividing and spreading of cancer cells.

Fourteen of the children in Study No. 6601 achieved remission for extended periods. Eric was not one of them. That said, the program underscored how effective using multiple drugs in combination could be.

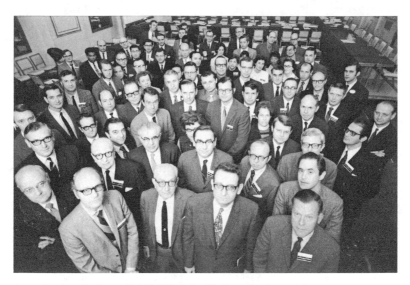

Acute Leukemia Group B (ALGB). John Vachon, *Look* magazine.

At the time, a leading cancer research group in the country, Acute Leukemia Group B, or ALGB, was headed by Dr. James Holland. This medical cooperative included many of the top doctors in the field—Donald Pinkel, Emil "Tom" Frei III, and Lucius Sinks. Shortly after being elected ALGB president in 1962, Holland moved the headquarters from suburban Washington to Buffalo. Even though that necessitated transferring only a few cartons of paper, it was indicative of the growing prominence of Roswell Park in the field of cancer research. In addition, Holland had the backing of C. Gordon Zubrod, who headed the Division of Cancer Treatment at the National Cancer Institute (NCI) outside Washington, D.C. Zubrod had secured a $5 million congressional grant to further the study of chemotherapy (using drugs such as vincristine and methotrexate in combinations) to battle cancer.

Zubrod, like many of the leukemia doctors, was well acquainted with personal loss. His mother had died when he was seven years old. An avid athlete growing up, Zubrod was forced to miss a year of high school due to a lung infection. He worked his way through Columbia Medical School as a waiter during the day and a library clerk at night. One summer, he worked for the Good Humor Ice Cream Company during his remaining off-hours.

Before coming to the NCI, Zubrod was on a medical team that explored ways to control malaria. The drugs deployed during this period—Atabrine and chloroquine—were crucial to the Allies' effort in the South Pacific during World War II. In 1946, Zubrod joined the staff of the Johns Hopkins University School of Medicine, where he participated with another group of scientists conducting research on bacterial pneumonia, the disease that had killed his mother.

Zubrod believed in teamwork, regardless of personality differences. He urged Holland in Buffalo and Tom Frei at the NCI to find a way to work in concert, even though they were at different hospitals, almost 400 miles apart. "Gordon was the grease that put Tom and me together," Holland said.

Under Holland's direction, the ALGB initiated more clinical trials in acute leukemia and met regularly, often in Washington. Between face-to-face meetings, the group found ways to continue to share information. "Of course, this was well before the Internet and cell phones," Dr. Donald Pinkel recalled. "But we still had regular phones and those early fax machines where the paper spun around on the drum. We found ways to stay in touch, to keep comparing notes, especially as things began to move forward with Jim in charge."

Despite having patients at multiple institutions, doctors followed a standardized protocol, which soon had as many as twenty-eight different categories. At first, the ALGB relied on data generated in the 1940s and 1950s by the NCI and such groups as

Sidney Farber's in Boston. But they soon broadened their research, and Pinkel said that discussions among Holland's growing group of leukemia doctors were usually frank and sometimes contentious. After a study Holland dearly wanted to be done was voted down, with several key members weighing in despite not attending the meeting in person, the chairman decided that nobody would "have a voice at the table unless you're an in-person participant."

The ALGB group documented that vincristine and prednisone could lead to significant periods of remission in leukemia patients when used together. Pinkel, Holland, and other doctors in this group soon agreed that more such cancer-fighting drugs, in larger dosages, should be deployed in more cases. The combination of vincristine and prednisone was followed up with 6-MP, methotrexate and a new drug, BCNU (bis-chloroethylnitrosourea), which some believed had the potential to cross the blood–brain interface. The ALGB doctors soon became convinced that such cancer drugs could be better used in various combinations—two, three, or even four or more at a time.

One drug often couldn't destroy all the cancer cells, Pinkel explained. "To really do the job, you needed a combination of agents, these chemotherapy drugs, many of which were just becoming available to us in the 1960s," he said. "Using them two, three, four at a time. That was a very fundamental observation and fundamental insight. It became key to our progress moving forward."

About this time, tests on mice indicated that large doses of methotrexate had the potential to be much more effective than limited doses of the same drug. That said, the growing number of chemotherapy drugs were considered dangerous poisons elsewhere in the medical community. How high could dosages be increased before the treatment potentially became as dangerous to the patient as the disease itself? That was the fine line Holland, Pinkel, and the others were beginning to walk.

Procedures needed to be so precise that my brother was weighed every time he visited Roswell Park, and extended stays at the hospital were carefully monitored. Study No. 6601 was broken into four groups of children, and it cannot be determined today which group Eric was in at the time. What we do know is that he began to recover. A decade after the procedure, nearly 30 percent of the patients in Study No. 6601 were still alive. Holland told me that Study No. 6601 "may have been the finest study done by our group."

On May 4, 1966, Eric officially went into remission. Compared with today, the term "remission" was never very definitive during my brother's short life. Decades later, I asked an expert in pharmacology to review my brother's flow chart of meds, the clinical trials he was a part of at Roswell Park.

"What I see is a patient who was always on some kind of chemotherapy medicine," she said. "He was never free of extensive care as you would expect a patient, especially one technically in remission, to be defined as today. That in itself underscores how fragile, how uncertain, all of this was back then."

IN SUMMER 1966, when Eric was first in remission, we began to sail as a family. While Dad already knew his way around a boat, the rest of us were rank beginners. Our first boat was a modest Penguin wooden dinghy. Only 11 feet long and less than five feet wide, the boat weighed about 150 pounds. Dad's plan was to sail it on the Erie Canal, which lay right across the road from our house in Lockport.

Shipping traffic on what used to be the main thoroughfare between Buffalo and the Hudson River, on the canal that had first opened up much of the Midwest to commerce, had dropped away to close to nothing by then. Those rare times when a barge did appear around the bend, we learned to hug the shoreline, bobbing in the wake until the larger vessel was well past us. If everything had gone according to plan, we could have sailed that Penguin on the canal for summers to come. But the dinghy's mast, the topping of a cat rig, was a smidge too tall for its own good. No matter how much we maneuvered the craft, leaning it well over to one side and then the other, we couldn't easily pass the mast underneath the steel-girder bridge less than a quarter mile west of home. It soon became apparent that we were cordoned off, unable to sail the Erie Canal for any real distance. Just to the west stood the Canal Road Bridge, and a mile or so in the opposite direction, around a gradual bend in the canal, lay the Orangeport Bridge. We were penned in, without enough space to really spread our sails.

Dad was a second-generation engineer who had been called home from graduate school in Ann Arbor to assist my Grandpa Lee when the family firm took off. Begun in a garage, the business eventually grew to more than fifty employees, working in a flat-roofed office that my father had designed, across the road from our house. At one point, as the oldest child, I was expected to join Wendel Engineers, maybe even take it over one day. But I could never get the necessary math right in my head, especially algebra.

Math would never be my forte. Instead I loved stories about pirates and knights, action heroes and cowboys, and so much more. Perhaps that's why of the two pursuits my father tried to teach me, engineering and sailing, we were able to make only half of the equation stick.

That said, I've always admired the diligence demonstrated by those in the sciences. How methodically they can work through a problem, pushing toward a solution. At first glance, civil engineers and leukemia doctors don't seem to have a lot in common. Yet they do share a dogged determination and a particular belief in the future. Where the rest of us may see only a roadblock or dead end, they can often gaze beyond it all, searching for the place on the far horizon where divergent clues may come together.

Because we were hemmed in on the Erie Canal, I began to accompany Dad on trips to Lake Ontario, a dozen or so miles down Route 78, past the small towns of Wrights Corners, Newfane, and Burt. Together we would walk to the end of the steel pier there, out to the small tower topped by the flashing red light, and survey the wide expanse of Lake Ontario. This was where Dad had first learned to sail, and soon enough we would know these waters too.

4

Under another set of circumstances, Donald Pinkel would have been my brother's supervising physician at Roswell Park. Even though the doctor was eventually forced to move hundreds of miles away from his hometown of Buffalo, Pinkel remained in contact with James Holland, Tom Frei, Emil "Jay" Freireich, and others in the effort against childhood cancer.

Pinkel's own health was in question when he returned home as the director of pediatrics at Roswell Park in 1956. (Part of his initial $9,000 salary came from funds provided by Mary Lasker, philanthropist and cancer advocate.) He moved his family into a modest two-story house on Woodward Avenue, only a few blocks from the zoo. He was twenty-nine years old, with four children underfoot and more on the way.

Any notion that his move back home would be a smooth one disappeared as quickly as the summertime temperatures. The winter weather caused pain in his limbs, the aftermath of a bout of polio, and the hours at his new post soon became long and arduous. Pinkel found himself at Roswell Park almost every day, and as soon as he parked his '49 DeSoto Coupe and went inside, the challenges usually mounted. The hospital in Buffalo had been in existence for decades, and sometimes Pinkel found Roswell Park too set in its ways for

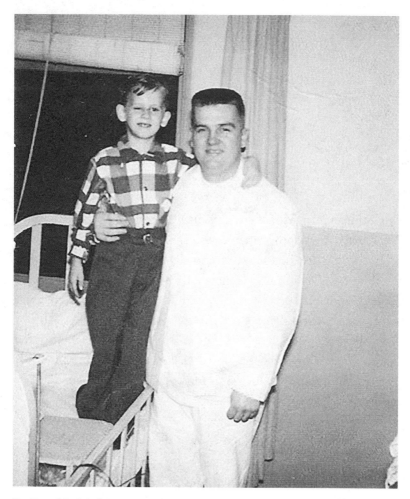

Dr. Donald Pinkel. Courtesy of the Pinkel family.

its own good. It fell to him to obtain money for more furniture, a playground, pajamas, and even diapers for the kids in his care. He brought in more doctors and nurses—ones more accustomed to treating children. In his spare time, he developed a pediatric cancer program, focusing on possible viral causes of leukemia.

Early in his time at Roswell Park, Pinkel lost three children to leukemia in a single day. As they died, he remained at their bedsides, talking to them in a hushed voice. Later on, back at home, he felt so depressed that he wondered how he could go back to work the next morning.

One of his mentors had warned Pinkel that he would be "throwing away his career" by staying in this field of medicine. After all, Pinkel was a highly regarded doctor with a growing family to take care of. He didn't have to hold to this path—taking on cancer with little support.

Still, as he sat alone at the kitchen table that night, Pinkel asked himself, "If these children and their parents can face this disease every day, what's wrong with me?" He realized that if he didn't care for them, few in the medical community would even try.

"The kids I was treating couldn't run from this and neither could their parents and family. So I decided I wouldn't either," he explained decades later. "If you saw a child drowning in a river, you wouldn't worry about how swift the current is or how deep the waters might be. You'd try to save him, wouldn't you?"

A fourth generation Buffalonian, Pinkel grew up idolizing his sister Ann Marie, who was thirteen years older than he was. After she became a student nurse at Mercy Hospital in south Buffalo, she would draw diagrams of the circulatory system on a small blackboard in the family home in Kenmore, New York. That's where Pinkel helped his friend Herby Morgan deliver the *Buffalo Evening News* and the *Kenmore Independent*, a local advertiser.

"There were always babies around," he said. "When my mother stopped having babies, my older sister began having babies. I used to do a lot of babysitting for them. I've always enjoyed being around kids."

Even though Pinkel became interested in medicine when he was five years old, back when his sister showed him what she had learned on the family blackboard, it would be some time before he took any formal courses in science. He attended Canisius High School, where he received a solid Jesuit education—Greek, Latin, and the classics—but, despite being a premed student with a double major in biology and chemistry, no science for several years. At the age of sixteen, he told the principal that he wanted to switch around his courses, delve into biology or physics. But the principal replied, "No, no—you must know why you are going to medicine first. You must read the humanities. You'll get plenty of science later on."

When he was in his senior year at Canisius High School, Pinkel joined the navy and was assigned to officer training at Cornell University in Ithaca, New York, about a three-hour drive away. There he became a medical officer and did premed training before going into the reserves and finishing his college education back home at Canisius College. Upon graduation, he began at the University of Buffalo School of Medicine. During his third year at the University of Buffalo, Pinkel was assigned to Children's Hospital in Buffalo, where he did his internship and residency.

"Children's Hospital was wonderful . . . ," Pinkel said. "They accepted everybody as patients. They didn't worry about whether they had money or not."

During his third year of residency, Pinkel took a course in cancer at E. J. Meyer Memorial Hospital, now Erie County Medical Center. Afterward, he began two- to three-week rotations at Roswell Park and won a grant from the Erie County American Cancer Society to study tumors. He was young man with a promising future, and that's when Dr. Mitchell Rubin first tried to intercede on his behalf. As chairman of pediatrics at Children's Hospital, Rubin was a formidable presence. He and Pinkel had crossed paths a few years earlier when Pinkel got permission to skip the last year of a rotating internship.

Rubin asked Pinkel, "Where does your heart lie? Where do you want to make your mark in the medical world?" When Pinkel replied that he was fascinated with cancer, especially in children, Rubin told him, "You're throwing away your career. We'll never figure it out."

When Pinkel refused to budge, Rubin told him to talk with Dr. George Moore, a talented young surgeon from the University of Minnesota, who had recently arrived in Buffalo to head up Roswell Park. At that point, there were no pediatric services at the research center. Yet Moore agreed with Pinkel that such services were sorely needed, and he promised to keep Pinkel in mind when the situation changed.

In the meantime, Pinkel took a commission in the army when he graduated from medical school. After reporting for active duty, he was assigned to the army hospital at Fort Devens, Massachusetts. There he was the sole pediatrician and the chief doctor when an epidemic of polio broke out. During the 1950s, Buffalo had seen several such outbreaks, and Pinkel believed that he was immune. Yet at Fort Devens he became severely exhausted, putting in long hours at the hospital. To the shock of everyone, the young doctor contracted polio too.

"It was touch and go whether I was going to survive or not," he said. "My respiratory function went down to a small fraction. . . . I remember going to sleep one night and I thought, 'Well, this it. I'm not going to wake up.' I thought I was going into an actual coma."

In the morning, Pinkel did awake—to a nurse sticking a cold thermometer into his mouth. He had lost feeling in much of his limbs and was transferred by ambulance to Murphy Army Hospital in Waltham, Massachusetts, fearful that the paralysis would become permanent. After being given a private room, Pinkel asked to be housed in the ward with the enlisted men returning from the Korean War because he missed being around people. In the ward, he went in the Hubbard tank, a device used for hydrotherapy, every morning and exercised in the afternoon. After six weeks, he began to regain use of his limbs.

One night, a medical officer asked Pinkel to examine a sick child. No other pediatrician was on duty. Even though he could barely sit up at the time, the young doctor was eager to help.

A nurse wheeled Pinkel over on a gurney, and he leaned over to examine the baby, who was severely dehydrated. Pinkel ordered an IV and instructed the nurses about the next round of care. As he did so, Pinkel thought, "That is the most wonderful thing that could have happened to me. I'm doing what I was meant to do."

This choice became a cornerstone of Pinkel's career. After practicing much of his career east of the Mississippi River (Boston, Buffalo, and Memphis), he now lives three hours south of San Francisco and teaches at California Polytechnic State University in San Luis Obispo. Despite being almost ninety years old, Pinkel still enjoys lecturing and being among students in the Biological Sciences Department. When discussing the old days, being on the frontier of cancer research, he sometimes nods his head, as if he is conducting an orchestra whose notes only he can hear.

"I've always believed that people, if given the resources, will always find the determination to take something on," he said, "even something that's considered impossible by some to overcome. Back when I was getting my start, people were ready to take on cancer and somebody had to lead the way. So each of us, in our own way, stepped in and tried to fill the void. And if that meant being called pirates and cowboys and other names that they heaped on us—so be it."

The Cancer Cowboys? I told Pinkel I liked the ring of that. How it captured this budding movement within medicine.

"It was just one of so many," he replied. "Other names they called us were much, much worse. Trust me."

Unfit for duty, Pinkel soon left the army and spent the better part of a year steadily moving from a wheelchair to leg braces to crutches, continuing his recovery at the Veterans' Administration (VA) hospital in West Roxbury, Massachusetts. During this time, he interviewed with Dr. Sidney Farber, a fellow Buffalonian and University of Buffalo Medical School alumnus, about working part-time at the Children's Cancer Research Foundation in Boston. A pediatric pathologist, Farber was having success with aminopterin, an aggressive antifolate, producing temporary remissions in children with leukemia. While Pinkel, Holland, and others would soon be using chemotherapy drugs increasingly in combination, many of the medications used to treat my brother and so many other kids like him can be traced back to this earlier period.

Farber was from Williamsville, New York, only 10 miles from where Pinkel had grown up. (Years later, the School of Pharmacy at the University of Buffalo would be named after Farber.) By the end of their conversation, Farber decided to take on Pinkel as "a half-time fellow," but only if the young doctor promised that he wouldn't allow work to interfere with his rehabilitation from polio. As a result, Pinkel began to do his therapy in the morning at the VA hospital, and afterward he drove directly to the clinic in Boston. Farber arranged that a parking spot be reserved for Pinkel by the front door.

Back in New York State, Governor Thomas Dewey, who had lost two members of his family to cancer, pushed for the expansion of the medical campus in Buffalo. George Moore began to gather more money from the state legislature in Albany, and a new building was soon under construction, with more doctors being hired. Pinkel took the train home to Buffalo to interview for the position as head of pediatrics.

"They had hoped to get a more senior person, but they couldn't find one, so I was it," he said. "There I was fresh out of the VA hospital, and a year of part-time experience in the field of cancer at Boston Children's with Dr. Farber."

In spring 1956, he took the job and moved his growing family into a home on Woodward Avenue, only a few blocks from Delaware Park. Pinkel's daughter, Becky, remembered that the family next door had thirteen kids, so there was always somebody to play with. One of Pinkel's brothers built the family a sandbox in the shape of a boat, and the Woodward home had a secret passageway upstairs. When Pinkel worked overnight at Roswell Park, he often stopped at Freddies Doughnuts, a local institution, on the way home, and his kids awoke to the treats on the kitchen table.

Occasionally, Pinkel's family visited at the hospital. Once they pulled into the back parking lot and saw a woman who had just died being transported away on a stretcher with a sheet over her entire body except her toes. The toes were painted a bright red—a color that daughter Becky would never forget. When she grew up, she never painted her nails red.

Many members of Pinkel's extended family had summer cottages across the Niagara River, along the Canadian shore of Lake Erie, and the doctor rented a rundown place for his family on Waverly Beach, not far from the Peace Bridge. By the end of the summer, when it was time to return to Woodward Avenue in Buffalo, Pinkel was reluctant to do so. Instead he found a brick farmhouse at Windmill Point, a mile or so from Lake Erie. It came with a run-down chicken coop and small pig barn. Yet with a new furnace and good insulation, the cottage at Windmill Point became the family's year-round residence for the rest of the doctor's time at Roswell Park.

The crunch of the car wheels on the gravel driveway meant Pinkel was home from the hospital, often with a notable person in medicine in tow. Dr. Robert Guthrie, who introduced the first newborn screening system in the United States, and Dr. Rita Levi-Montalcini, the Nobel Prize winner, were among those who visited Windmill Point. One time Pinkel came home so late from the hospital that he had to throw snowballs at the bedroom windows to summon somebody to let him in; after that, the front door remained unlocked.

"My dad's patients nearly always died, at least early on," Becky Pinkel said. "So there were times when he would come home to our house in Canada and sit on the porch at night and look out on those fields. Just alone with his thoughts.

"I remember him telling me one night about how some parents dropped off their child at Roswell Park because they could not stand to see him suffer anymore. Everybody expected this one child to die and he soon did. My dad and his staff, of course, had no choice but to watch and to try and do the best that they could."

5

"Wait until you see it," Dad said as we turned off Route 18, the main drag through the village of Youngstown, New York. "It is a gorgeous boat."

He was behind the wheel as we headed down Water Street, the steep one-way loop toward the Niagara River. All of us kids were wedged in the back of the Buick station wagon, and we leaned forward, eager for a better look, as more and more of the cobalt-blue waters below came into view. On the other side of the river, we saw flags flying, the British Union Jack, atop a stockade-style fort, Fort George. That vision, like something from a storybook, disappeared from view as we rolled closer to the river, which now took up more and more of the frame until we parked alongside an emerald-green lawn that extended right to the water's edge.

Because the Penguin's mast was too tall to pass under the steel-girder bridges crossing the Erie Canal, we had started to spend more time at Lake Ontario, visiting the small harbors that dot the southern rim between the Niagara River and Rochester. Such places as Youngstown, Wilson, and Olcott may have been sleepy towns on the map, but they all opened onto this wide expanse of water; and they were places my father knew, where he had first learned to sail, and now he had returned to this region with a boat of his own.

Soon we were out of the car, walking across the freshly cut grass, all of us quiet as Dad gestured toward the public dock. Out on the river, sailboats varying greatly in size and rigging configuration were tied to orange buoys, riding the strong current, their bows pointed upstream, where Niagara Falls itself roared to life 20 miles away.

At the far end of the wharf, a launch with a loud motor was preparing to shove off. Filling the open area in the back were people, with canvas bags full of groceries and ice, eager to be carried out to one of the sailboats standing like sentries in the neat mooring rows. We would soon learn that the launch was nicknamed the Bum Boat and that its chief purpose was to shepherd people back and forth between the mainland and their particular craft.

Three other boats, all sailboats, were tied to the Youngstown Yacht Club public dock that afternoon. One was 30 feet or longer in length, and its deck was covered in ropes and sail bags. It was easy to imagine that it had returned from a long voyage somewhere out on Lake Ontario, which we could glimpse around the last bend downriver.

Just past it, bobbing in the water along the wooden dock, was a smaller sailboat with dark-blue fiberglass so bright and new that the glare caused me to squint. Although the mast was in place and the rigging set, compared to the bigger boat it had far fewer ropes, as if it was missing several key pieces.

"We're still waiting on the blocks," Dad said. "Maybe some bigger winches too."

None of us knew what he was talking about.

"They tell me it will be good to go by next weekend," Dad continued. "We'll be able to go out for a sail."

"So this is our boat now?" Susan asked.

"Done deal," Dad told us. "C'mon, there's no law against us getting on board today. Taking a look around to see what it will be like."

He stepped down from the wharf and into the small cockpit. He held out his hand for my mother, and once she was on board, the rest of us followed. All of us crowded into the cockpit, trying not to bump into the stick tiller that steered the strange craft. Eric and Bryan were both in life jackets, and I remember thinking that, even though I was the oldest and best swimmer in the bunch, I wouldn't have minded wearing a life jacket that day too. Despite the laughter and excited conversation from the other boaters around us, the ones who were old hands at navigating the Niagara River and Lake Ontario, we remained quiet, not sure what kind of world we had fallen into.

Dad began to tell us about the boat, our new boat. Although most of it didn't stick that afternoon, we would soon know as much about this craft as we would a member of the family. For we now owned a Shark 24, the class of boat originally designed by George Hinterhoeller and built across the Niagara River in Canada. Our boat was 24 feet long and 6 feet 10 inches at the beam, or its widest area across. It came with two sails, a mainsail that flew from the mast and a smaller jig that streamed back from the front forestay.

"It's a popular class of boat," Dad said. "You'll find hundreds of them on the Great Lakes. There's one now."

He pointed downriver, to where the Niagara River emptied into Lake Ontario. We shaded our eyes and gazed in that direction, and sure enough, there was a Shark sailboat, with both sails up, making good progress upwind. From a distance, it seemed to be a fast boat, certainly a far cry from sailing the Penguin on the Erie Canal.

The following weekend, Dad began to teach us about the wind—this invisible force that can shift and change direction in a heartbeat. "It never stays the same," he told us. "And you cannot go straight into it. At least not in a sailboat."

Motorboats were termed "stink potters" and considered a level or two below boats that used the wind for forward propulsion. If you could picture what the wind was doing, not only acknowledge its power but harness its frequent gusts, it could take you anywhere on the water.

Dad soon hung short strands of yarn to the metal wires, or shrouds, coming down from the mast that attached at the hull halfway between the bow and the stern. At amidships, we were told, and we were expected to learn such nautical terms. A rope, for example, was always called "a line" out on the water. "Rope" was a term used by landlubbers, and there was nothing worse than being viewed as a landlubber in a sailing world.

We watched as Dad tied the pieces of yarn to the strings of metal. He called them "telltales" and "who-whos," both terms used within the sailing community. Whatever they were called, the ribbons of yarn soon billowed out, showing us the direction of the wind. Within weeks, we became as excited as he did when the wind gusted, roughing the water's surface. For the new scallops and divots, appearing as a darker hue, sometimes called cat's paws, were sure signs that more wind, at least a momentary gust, was coming our way.

Before we learned to sail and moved to Olcott for the summers, the Erie Canal had been our pathway into a larger world. As long as we stuck to the towpath, Mom would let us older kids bike to a friend's house without a lift in the family wagon. We would call when we got there, and under such arrangements, we secured what any kid really desires—some measure of freedom and a way to get into trouble.

The summer before we moved to the lake for the season, Steve MacEvoy and I biked down to the Girl Scout camp. The front entrance was at Canal Road, just up from the intersection with Route 31 and the drive-in that once stood there. But there was a back entrance that Steve had discovered off the canal towpath. We ditched our bikes in the bushes and hiked into the camp one morning.

"Stay low," Steve said. "We can't let anybody see us."

With him leading the way, we headed down a ravine, deeper into the campground. Out before us, we saw rows of young women in white T-shirts and green shorts. They were doing jumping jacks and calisthenics as three older girls barked out the count. I remember Steve and I were eleven, maybe twelve years old at the time.

Creeping closer, angling for a better look, I fell over a small log. On the parade grounds, the jumping jacks stopped.

"Boys," somebody shouted, and with that, Steve and I ran as fast as we could back down and up to the ravine, coming out again on the towpath. We fished our bikes out of the bushes where we had stashed them and pedaled as fast as we could for home.

"Don't you come back here," one of the counselors shouted as Steve and I pedaled away.

Joyce Carol Oates, among the most prolific writers of our time, has set many of her stories in Lockport and the surrounding area. *Little Bird of Heaven; Because It Is Bitter, and Because It Is My Heart;* and *We Were the Mulvaneys* come to mind.

I met Oates once, and we discussed our hometown. She had written that the region suggests "a more innocent time imagined by Thornton Wilder or Edward Hopper, appropriated now by movie director David Lynch: the slightly sinister, surreal yet disarmingly 'normal'-seeming atmosphere of a quintessential American town trapped in a sort of spell or enchantment."

Oates was raised in a farmhouse near Transit Road, an area that has been transformed in recent years from a two-lane road running through small towns and farmland to a multilane highway that sweeps southward to the interstate encircling much of Buffalo. I'd read that she often took the city bus to the Lockport Public Library on East Avenue and surveyed the old locks on the Erie Canal, the "Flight of Five," from the Exchange Street Bridge.

"Where in Lockport did you grow up?" she asked, and I told her about the family farmhouse across the road from the Erie Canal, a few miles past Lowertown and the Wide Waters Marina.

"I know exactly where that is," she said.

"But we spent our summers down at Olcott," I added. "We lived year-round on Canal Road and I went to high school in Middleport."

Oates nodded in recognition. "Oh, that's the real Lockport," she said.

Eudora Welty once wrote that place in any story needs to be "named, identified, concrete, exact, and exacting." Without it, Welty maintained, "every story would be another story, and unrecognizable as art, if it took up its characters and plot and happened somewhere else. Imagine *Swann's Way* laid in London, or *The Magic Mountain* in Spain, or *Green Mansions* in the Black Forest. . . . From the dawn of man's imagination, place has enshrined the spirit; as soon as man stopped wandering and stood still and looked about him, he found a god in that place; and from then on, that was where the god abided and spoke from if ever he spoke."

After grade school, I regularly ran on the towpath of the Erie Canal. Workouts for the school track and cross-country teams were rarely talked about in terms or miles or time, the usual barometers of such drills. Instead, the coaches told us to run to the lift bridge in the center of Middleport and cross over to the dirt banks of the Erie, where it was easy to imagine we were following in the path of the packet boats pulled by a mule named Sal. (Yes, we had to learn the words to that folk song standby, "Low Bridge, Everybody Down," in grade school.) We would usually run one or two bridges up the Erie Canal before crossing at one of the steel-girder bridges that sweep high up from either bank, with the honeycomb-grid flooring, where we could see right through all the way down to the blue-gray waters below. From there, we would double back to school.

My best friend, John Douglas, lived between the bridges at Bolton and Telegraph Roads. On Fridays, I'd sometimes get off the bus at his house, and my father would pick me up after dinner. John's house was one of those rambling homesteads that always seems to have some kind of construction project going on—plumbing work in the kitchen, the hood up on another vehicle in the driveway. A barn with peeling red paint stood past the driveway, and that's where I first fired a BB gun. (We weren't allowed to have any firearms at our house.) And it was at John's that we gathered for Halloween. By then, I had graduated in my mind from trick or treat in Lockport at my grandparents' place, where the redbrick lanes were lined with streetlights and almost every house handed out candy, to something more reckless. At least that's what we told ourselves by that first year of junior high, when we regularly rode the bus home from Middleport. All along the Erie Canal, about a day's walk apart, such small towns as Gasport, Medina, and Spencerport were strung like pearls on a necklace. Middleport lies approximately halfway between Buffalo and Rochester.

We gathered for Halloween at John's on a chilly, windy night with no intention of collecting any candy. Instead we were armed with several rolls of toilet paper each—intent on transforming telephone poles, trees, and perhaps even somebody else's house into a spectacle of white tendrils that Salvador Dalí might appreciate.

Walking along Slayton Settlement Road, toward the canal, we set on the last telephone pole before the road narrowed and led up to the girder bridge and the intersection with Telegraph Road on the other side. Time and again, we threw the rolls into the air, letting them drape over the wires and snake down the pole itself until it was recast in ghostly webbing. John absolutely loved such fun. While the rest of us were afraid of getting caught, he didn't seem to care. Always the first to run out of toilet paper, he would beg for more from the rest of us. Despite the cold night, he led us to the towpath afterward, and we skipped stones in the canal, unable to see how many times each stone skimmed across the water in the darkness. The occasional car would pass over the Telegraph Road Bridge high above us, and we laughed like hyenas as it braked, briefly taking in the mess we had created in the telephone wires, before roaring on.

For our first summer on the water, *Ibeecha* was moored in the long lines of boats tethered to orange buoys off the Youngstown Yacht Club. With five kids in tow and all our gear, it took two or more trips aboard the Bum Boat to get everything shipshape and ready to cast off. We were burning daylight, time that we could be on the water, Dad decided. He began to search for a better situation and soon located dock space in Olcott, where he had learned to sail. A short walk from the gravel parking lot to an array of docks called the "Pig Pen" put us on the water so much sooner.

I was on board, with a few of Dad's buddies, when we officially sailed the Shark out the entrance to the Niagara River and took a wide starboard turn and headed along the southern shore of Lake Ontario. There wasn't much wind that afternoon, and it was dusk by the time we sighted the flashing red light that marked the entrance to Olcott's small harbor. Dousing the sails and starting the Evinrude outboard motor, it became a short ride in from the big lake, past the yacht club, where the sound of laughter and conversation carried easily across the water.

We found our new slip, the place where we would soon spend more and more of our summers. After we stored the sails and locked up the boat, we walked in single file toward the parking lot and our rides back home. In the darkness, the lights of the hamlet's few houses and the yacht club farther up the channel illuminated the calm waters inside the pair of breakwalls. Beyond the red light at the end of the left-hand-side pier, everything in the lake had already fallen into darkness. Only the sounds of the wind in the treetops and the waves crashing against the shore reached us now.

6

In September 1966, Eric came down with a severe infection, with a sore throat and achiness in the joints. He was put on antibiotics for a week, which began to clear things up, but he wasn't able to continue in Study No. 6601. Officially he had relapsed, and a new round of chemotherapy drugs—prednisone and 6-MP—was ordered. By mid-November, Eric was healthy enough to be enrolled in a new clinical trial, No. 6608.

Early trials had shown that 6-mercaptopurine, or 6-MP, could inhibit tumors and perhaps slow the growth of cancer cells in patients with acute leukemia. For some reason, 6-MP worked better in children than in adult leukemia patients. Warning labels for 6-MP emphasize that this "is a potent drug. It should not be used unless [there is] a diagnosis of acute lymphatic leukemia. . . ." The long list of side effects includes nausea, darkening of the skin, and hair loss.

Cancer cells, especially if they are dividing and multiplying, can bring 6-MP into the process. Imagine a locomotive train pulling out of the station, already picking up speed. This scenario is like the cancer cells as they begin another cycle of dividing and multiplying and growing, becoming more dangerous, more formidable. If 6-MP can become a part of this process, one of the last passengers, running along the platform and jumping aboard as the train leaves the station, the cancer doesn't realize it. Pack enough 6-MP on board, and these rogue passengers can slow the train down, even derail this round of the cancer, buying more time for the doctors and researchers.

In the mid-1960s, when my brother was diagnosed, the average person couldn't wrap his mind around the word "leukemia" and the fledgling treatments for it. The doctors involved in this effort were rarely certain of the timing, frequency, duration, or dosage of treatments. Deploying drugs like 6-MP sounded like something out of science fiction, and as a result, the doctors were often criticized by their peers.

"To many in the medical establishment, we were seen as reckless or even irresponsible," Dr. Jerry Yates said. "That resulted in many of the names that they called us—killers, poison pushers, renegades, pirates, cowboys."

Of course, Eric knew nothing of such debates within the medical community. Still, he seemed to understand how precarious life's balance had become for him. Once when Mom was driving him home from another round of treatments at Roswell Park, he sat in the back seat, smiling as the passing scenery faded from city to suburb as they headed north to Millersport Highway and on to Transit Road. Soon they would be back at home on Canal Road.

"Nothing could be finer," he said, almost humming to himself, "than riding in a car."

Often on the way home, the two of them stopped at Gleason's, a restaurant in the Boulevard Mall. No matter what he ordered, Eric would finish the meal off with lemon meringue pie. For Mom, his favorite dessert became a sign of the times. "The sweet meringue atop the sour tang of lemon and the piecrust holding the whole thing together," she said. "That there might be a solution to this great puzzle."

The combination of 6-MP and prednisone stabilized my brother's condition. By mid-December, Eric was well enough to be home with us for Christmas. That was always a grand holiday in our household because we actually celebrated the day twice. In the morning, we awoke and raced downstairs to see what Santa had left under the tree at our home on Canal Road. The usual mayhem would ensue, with perhaps the topper coming when my brother Bryan, who was a year younger than Eric, drove his new go-cart down the cellar steps.

By mid-afternoon, we made ourselves presentable enough to head into town, Lockport itself, for a second round of gift opening and Christmas dinner at my grandparents' house on Morrow Avenue. Their three-bedroom colonial, with a separate garage in back, where my grandfather had first opened his survey and engineering business, had once stood on the outskirts of town. Over the years, the growth of the town had engulfed it, with wide sidewalks and kids our own age to play with. I always loved visiting Morrow Avenue, as my grandmother was a great cook—pies and bread from scratch and pot roasts on Sundays—and we could always get a game of cowboys and Indians or touch football going. In this part of the world, a new contest often began when the Wendels showed up, with three or more of us ready to play.

My parents agreed that if Eric remained healthy enough, he would begin kindergarten at Gasport Elementary in the fall. With Mom needing to spend more time with him at Roswell Park, the rest of us had to step up. My family was never one for elaborate explanations. In all the years Eric was sick, we knew he was in bad shape, that he could possibly die, but I don't remember us ever having a conversation around the dinner table, where everything was detailed or fully explained to us. It just wasn't my parents' way.

Their focus was on living fully in this day and the next and the one after that. The emphasis became on the process, the implementation, the action itself. That's when we were at our best as a family. As a result, we began to take longer and longer sailing trips across open water. Perhaps this was the only way my parents, especially my father, could deal with things.

Decades later, when my own children were nearly adults, I came across Wade Davis's book *Into the Silence: The Great War, Mallory, and the Conquest of Everest.* It details the initial British attempts at reaching the summit of Mount Everest in the 1920s and how the British came to Tibet so gung ho and driven to reach the top of the world's highest peak. It was a mind-set that completely flummoxed the locals. After all, the Tibetans asked, "can't we be happy just gazing upon such majestic snowcapped peaks? Why should one feel we have to climb them, too?"

The British climbers never fully answered such questions. The best they could come up with was George Mallory's famous quip: "Because it's there." Yet when somebody considers the bigger picture, the Everest campaigns had to be made. The British, along with most of Europe, had just fought World War I. The trench warfare, rapid-fire machine guns, barbed wire, and mustard gas were a nightmare for an entire continent, a whole generation. The British climbers were drawn to try and rise above it all, to attempt to climb the highest peak in the world, to move into the silence.

In our way, my family was able to temporarily escape the clamor and discord too. Though we weren't climbing Mount Everest, a wide horizon of water has always calmed my father. And even though Dad never came out and said it, he had to believe that it would help the rest of us too.

When I told Donald Pinkel about those family voyages, how we became sailors during the summers when Eric was sick, sailing across that vast inland sea, he seemed to understand.

"That was your family's reaction to this immense challenge," he said. "Maybe it's like my family moving to a cottage on Lake Erie, making it our year-round home. How we tried, in our own particular ways, to cope with the enormity of it all."

7

One July afternoon, we were sailing along the southern U.S. shore, heading toward the entrance to the Niagara River. Beyond that lies the Welland Canal, which connects Lake Erie to Lake Ontario for commercial shipping traffic. For much of its history, Ontario was the forgotten Great Lake. Freighters and cargo boats coming from the west, through the other four lakes—Superior, Michigan, Huron, and Erie—needed to transfer their goods and raw materials at Buffalo onto smaller packet boats for the passage farther east on the Erie Canal. It wasn't until 1959, when the St. Lawrence Seaway opened to deep-water shipping, that freighters large enough to navigate the oceans began to move through Lake Ontario.

On this day, we were still getting used to the genoa jib, the sail that took up much of the foredeck and extended well back from the top of the mast, almost to the cockpit. It had slid off the track when pulled upward by the halyard, and Dad took my brother Chris forward of the mast to fix it. The detail was supposed to be a short one—done so we could turn and begin a longer tack farther out onto the lake. As Dad and Chris worked away, the sail blocked their vision.

"We should turn soon," I said, glancing around us.

I was at the helm, and while no other vessels were in the immediate vicinity, I could see one lake freighter and then another, nothing more than low-slung shadows right now, approaching the nearby shipping lanes.

"In a minute," Dad replied. He was on one knee, pliers in hand. "We need to get this done first."

That was how things remained until a long, gray-hulled freighter came into focus, making a graceful pass toward the entrance to the Welland Canal.

"There's a freighter off to our left," I told Dad.

"You mean port," said my sister Susan. Back then she had grasped the nautical lingo better than I had.

"We have time," Dad replied, without looking.

He and Chris remained shielded by our own sail. Only the rest of us, farther back in the cockpit, could see the freighter growing ever larger as it began to bear down on us. Sometimes it's amazing how fast something so huge—five stories or taller above the waterline—can move. Take a look and it's somewhere off in the distance, nothing to really worry about. Look again and it's already here, taking up more and more of your world in a hurry.

"Dad, it's getting closer," I called out. "We need to come around."

Mom sat in the cockpit and followed my gaze to the approaching freighter, where white waves were now visible coming off its square bow.

"Dad?" I asked, but he waved me off, still hard at work on the sail.

"We need to turn," I told mother.

"Peter," she said.

"I said, just a minute," Dad replied. "We're almost finished—"

Mom glanced around, making sure that Eric and Bryan had life jackets on, and I reached into the lazarette, a small compartment in the back of the boat, rummaging around for one for myself.

"Dad, we need to turn—now."

"I told you, just a minute," Dad answered.

With that the sail edge finally loosened, and the sheet of off-white Dacron, which had been concealing our rapidly deteriorating situation from my father, cascaded in a whoosh down to the deck. Dad and Chris gathered up the sail, keeping it from tumbling into the water. Then they gazed up to see the lake freighter, which now resembled a floating building, hovering over the top of us. We were so close that faces were visible in the portholes, and more sailors peered over the rail down on us.

"Hard-a-lee, hard-a-lee!" Dad yelled as he ran back to the cockpit.

I had already begun to tack away. Susan commandeered the mainsail, keeping it from fluttering in the wind for long and trimming it tight once we finished the maneuver.

"Hold on," Dad warned, and a moment later, the set of huge waves created by the freighter's wake crashed into us. Chris kept himself from going over the side by hanging on to the forestay and lifelines. Somehow he kept the sail from going over the side too. Dad gathered up the smaller kids in a big bear hug as they slid together across the cockpit floor. Everyone hung on for dear life until the freighter was far to our stern, continuing the sweeping turn toward the Welland Canal.

The irony was that Dad always did his due diligence before going out on the water. He listened to weather reports from multiple cities, purchased a shortwave radio so he could gather more information about approaching cold fronts, and studied radar maps of the possible storms when they became available. When I look back on that close call, the freighter coming into view, as intent on destruction and ill will as any life-threatening disease, I'm reminded that the best of tools and instructions can only do so much. Keeping an eye on the strips of yarn sewn along the leading edge of the sail or the weather vane atop the mast, staying focused on the horizon in rough seas, being cognizant of the compass heading on a foggy day—all of it sometimes doesn't do a lick of good. As my brother Eric knew better than any of us, a predicament that dissolves into a crisis can be like a perplexing, infuriating puzzle. Once the clock begins ticking down, the only question that remains is, how fast can you find a solution? How fast can you run to the top of the stairs and dare to sing out, "Ibeecha"?

8

Kindred spirits can usually be found if one stops long enough to listen to the echoes of yesteryear. The Pinkels' first family home was only a few blocks away from Delaware Park in Buffalo. Pinkel knew about the national tragedy that had unfolded on those grounds in 1901, that Roswell Park had been a renowned, somewhat star-crossed doctor long before becoming the name of a world-famous cancer research hospital.

Born in Pomfret, Connecticut, Roswell Park was only two years old when his mother died. Raised by his father and his uncle, Park received his B.A. in 1872 from Racine College in Wisconsin and graduated with high honors from Northwestern in 1878. During his residency at Cook County Hospital in Chicago, he became well versed in the treatment of gunshot wounds. In a cruel twist, he wasn't able to exhibit such expertise when it mattered most.

Park was appointed the chair of surgery at the Medical Department of Buffalo in 1883. Even though he was initially denied financial assistance by the state, he eventually secured the necessary funding to open the first hospital in the world dedicated to cancer research. When the Pan-American Exposition began its six-month run in Buffalo in 1901, Park was appointed the medical director and ranking surgeon of the event.

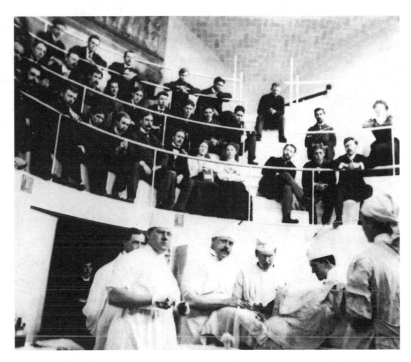

Dr. Roswell Park (center) operates in front of a packed gallery in Buffalo. Courtesy of the Dr. Roswell Park Biographical File, University Archives, University at Buffalo, the State University of New York.

On September 6, 1901, President William McKinley paid a visit to western New York. McKinley had easily won reelection in 1900 and enjoyed mingling with his admirers. On this hot afternoon, the fifty-eight-year-old president dismissed the warnings of his security detail and shook hands for several hours in the Temple of Music, a redbrick hall on the exposition grounds in Delaware Park. As the event drew to a close, a twenty-eight-year-old man in a dark suit approached McKinley. The man had waited more than two hours to greet the president, and his right hand was curiously wrapped in a handkerchief. Noticing the apparent injury,

McKinley reached out to shake the man's left hand. That's when Leon Czolgosz, a self-proclaimed anarchist, took another step forward and fired two shots from a .32-caliber Iver Johnson revolver that was concealed by the handkerchief in his hand. One bullet caused only a superficial wound, but the other struck the president in the abdomen, and McKinley soon lost consciousness.

At the time of the shooting, Roswell Park was almost 30 miles away performing an operation in Niagara Falls, New York. When a messenger burst in with news of the assassination attempt, Park hurried to finish the procedure but refused to leave until everything was complete. It was late afternoon by the time Park arrived at the exposition grounds in Buffalo. There he found a makeshift operating room with Dr. Matthew Mann, chairman of obstetrics and gynecology at the University of Buffalo, in charge. Even though Park was by far the more experienced surgeon, he refused to take over and only advised Mann. That decision would haunt Park for the rest of his life.

Operating conditions were far from ideal that day. President McKinley was in an ether-induced sleep, and a mirror was used to reflect the sun's rays, giving Mann slightly more light to operate. As a crowd gathered outside, an official statement was released at 7 p.m. It detailed McKinley's injuries and that the second bullet hadn't been found. What it failed to mention was that Mann had decided not to drain the wound in the president's abdomen. Only a few weeks earlier (or later—accounts differ), Park had saved a local woman who had shot herself twice in the abdomen with a pistol—an apparent suicide attempt. In that case, "posterior and anterior drainage" was deployed, and the woman made a full recovery.

At first, it appeared that McKinley would recover too. Within seventy-two hours, he was sitting up in bed, enjoying toast and coffee. Vice President Teddy Roosevelt was so reassured that he left Buffalo for a family vacation in the Adirondacks. Within days, however, McKinley's condition steadily worsened. Forty years before penicillin was available, the president was suffering from gangrene, which had formed along the pathway of the second bullet. In the early morning hours of September 14, he died among a small group of family and friends, including Park.

More than a century later, a small exhibit documenting these events can be seen inside the doors of the new Roswell Park hospital on the growing medical campus in downtown Buffalo. My brother's old hospital is gone, and many of his doctors no longer call western New York home. That said, Pinkel, Holland, and others remember Roswell Park, the doctor, as the main character in a cautionary tale of what can happen when a doctor becomes so caught up with protocol and convention that he cannot find a way to do everything he can to save his patient

9

With the aid of a cane, Dr. Lucius Sinks moved briskly through the dining room at the Boar's Head Inn in Charlottesville, Virginia. At eighty-two, he remained a formidable presence, with thick white hair, dark eyes, and a wry smile.

"So you made it down from D.C.?" he asked after taking the seat across the table.

It had taken me several months to discover that Sinks lived only a few hours away from me. I knew that if my search was going to have any real understanding and purpose, I needed to talk with the chief cancer research pediatrician, the top doctor in that wing of the hospital during the time my brother was at Roswell Park. What I didn't expect was that our lunchtime gatherings would become a regular occurrence that both of us seemed to enjoy.

My plan had been to wait until later in that initial conversation, bide my time, at least a bit. But I couldn't resist. Too soon I asked Sinks if he remembered my brother, his patient from almost four decades ago.

Sinks slowly shook his head. "I've thought a lot about it since you first contacted me," he replied. "But you have to remember that I saw a lot of children during my years at Roswell Park."

He stopped, as if to consider my question again. "Right now, I'm afraid not," the doctor said. "But let's just talk a while. See what the two of us can piece together."

We placed our orders and, around us, the restaurant filled with the buzz of noontime conversation. I listened as Sinks began to peel back the years, detailing how Roswell Park, St. Jude in Memphis, MD Anderson in Houston, the Dana-Farber Institute in Boston, and the National Cancer Institute outside of Washington, D.C., were among the few hospitals that came together in the early effort against childhood leukemia.

"Impressive institutions—no doubt," he said. "But there weren't many others back then, in the '60s. It's just the way things were when your brother came to us. The odds certainly weren't in our favor back in those days. But I suspect that you'll find that most of us who ended up in this line of work were already used to long odds."

As a boy, Sinks grew up on the North Shore of Boston. In the winters, skating and playing hockey became one of his first passions. When the marshland near his home in Marblehead froze, he became adept at dodging between the cattails and tall grasses and somehow keeping control of the puck. He was solidly built and believes that he would have excelled in the game if his family had stayed in the Boston area.

When Sinks was thirteen years old, his father, Allen, suffered a brain aneurysm. Sinks was away at summer camp on Sebago Lake in Maine when it occurred, and his father died within a few days. Today a CAT scan could have located the slight rupture in the brain, and a relatively simple procedure could have saved his life. That was far from the case in 1944.

Even though Anna Batchelder Sinks had deep roots in New England, she decided to move her children to Columbus, Ohio, where her husband's side of the family had even stronger ties and certainly more wealth. Allen G. Thurman, Lucius's great-great-grandfather, had served in the Senate for twelve years and was on the presidential ticket with Grover Cleveland in 1888, narrowly losing to Benjamin Harrison. Thurman was known for carrying a large red handkerchief that he waved to cheering crowds at political rallies. Another of Sinks's relatives, William Allen, had been governor of Ohio and also served in Congress. His statue represented Ohio in the National Statuary Collection on Capitol Hill for 129 years. (In 2016, it was replaced with a statue of Thomas Edison.) George Sinks, Lucius's great-grandfather, was a bank president in Columbus for two decades, and Frederick Sinks, his grandfather, was a prominent lawyer in town and an early supporter of the Columbus Academy, a private school in nearby Gahanna, Ohio. That's where Lucius and his younger brothers soon enrolled after their father's death. Founded in 1911, the academy was an all-boys school until 1991.

After graduating from the Columbus Academy, Sinks headed to Yale, where his parents had met years before, and in 1953, he became one of the first students there to earn a B.S. in biophysics. After a professor told him he wasn't smart enough to pursue a Ph.D., Sinks went into medicine. He did his residency at Columbus Children's Hospital and then served in the air force. Stationed at the Royal Air Force Mildenhall base in eastern England, where scenes for the movie *Twelve O'Clock High* had been filmed, Sinks began to spend his off-hours at Cambridge University.

"I walked in cold and eventually wormed my way into [Dr. Frank G. J.] Hayhoe's department," Sinks said. "Hayhoe was a stiff-upper-lip Brit and I remember that he didn't think that much of my writing skills. That said, I learned a great deal from him. He was one of the top experts in leukemia research on either side of the pond."

Sinks was in the air force from 1958 to 1961, and soon afterward, he won a fellowship from the National Cancer Institute, which gave him the opportunity to be a junior fellow under Hayhoe at Cambridge. At the time, doctors were meticulously studying cyto-chemical stains under a microscope, trying to pinpoint particular leukemia cells and their specific cell cycles.

"It was real grunt work," Sinks said. "But it helped us understand more about the cycles and the prolific rates of leukemia. This al-lowed us to be more specific in our treatments, which is something that I was really involved with when I came to Buffalo."

In 1966, Sinks arrived in Buffalo, following in Pinkel's footsteps as the Roswell Park director of pediatrics.

"A lot of academic people were against what we were trying to do," Sinks continued. "They really didn't understand some of the methods we were beginning to deploy against the cancer and, as a result, there was considerable resistance. Some pediatricians even refused to refer their kids to us. Some of them couldn't accept what we were doing. Not one iota of it."

I wondered if Sinks's teachers and mentors had advised him to focus on another line of medicine, if they had been like Donald Pinkel's mentor: urging him to steer away from a career in child-hood leukemia.

"To be honest, some did. They thought they were doing me a favor," Sinks said. "But I guess my problem was that I always liked working with kids the best. You see, kids always tell you how they feel. They don't pull any punches. I soon came to appreciate that kind of honesty. When you think about it, it's pretty unusual in the world."

As we began to leave, Sinks asked me to send him a photo of Eric. "Something to spark my memory," he said.

After the two-hour drive back to my home in northern Vir-ginia, I emailed him one of the few family photos I have from that time. In it, the entire Wendel family is lined up for the camera, with my parents and little sister Amy up front and the rest of us standing in a row of five behind them. My brother Eric is second from the left. Despite having lost his hair, due to another round of chemotherapy, he had a thin, knowing smile on his face.

Eric was the fairest, in terms of complexion and hair color, of any of us. Although Bryan and Amy sported blond curls soon after being born, those locks eventually faded toward the dark hair the rest of us had. In the summer, after spending time on the water, the rest of us quickly grew tanned from the bright sun. "As brown as Indians," my Grandma Mimi said. All of us, that is, except Eric.

Out on the water, Mom made sure her son wore a wide-brimmed hat and slathered on the sunblock to keep his face, arms, and legs from becoming red and inflamed. While his stature and even body type seemed to swell or shrink, depending on the meds he was on, his eyes and expressions never really changed that much. His alert eyes kept tabs on everything around him. When he smiled, it wasn't all teeth and giggles like the rest of us. His grin was thin, with something always held in reserve. As if he somehow knew better.

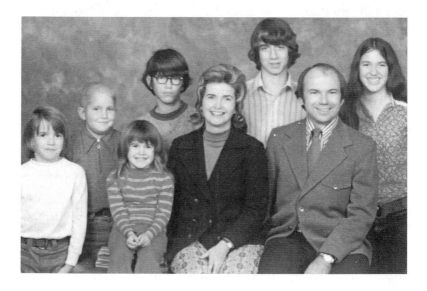

Despite missing school due to the treatments at Roswell Park, Eric maintained high grades, especially in math and science. Unlike me, he had the makings of an engineer.

A few days after our lunch in Charlottesville, Sinks emailed that the photo had helped him turn back the clock, at least a little bit. While he still couldn't place my brother, he remembered my mother, who somehow remained upbeat, optimistic, and determined despite the myriad of medical procedures Eric faced.

"Unfortunately, your brother fell into the pattern of so many children in our care," Sinks wrote. "We could help them survive, often longer than expected, but it took some luck and real magic for those like your brother to live anything like a normal life."

10

By the late 1960s, the median survival rate for children with acute lymphoblastic leukemia had risen to almost two years. During this period, Dr. James Holland gave a landmark report at a meeting of the American Association for Cancer Research at the Bellevue-Stratford Hotel in Philadelphia. Holland told the audience that intensive drug treatments administered to children, using multiple chemotherapy drugs at the same time, had resulted in "periods of six months or more in which the disease symptoms were absent."

By now, Eric was on daunomycin coupled with prednisone. Doctors and nurses using this form of chemotherapy needed to be extremely careful because the drug could cause blistering if it came into direct contact with human tissue. Classified as an antitumor antibiotic, it came from the soil fungus *Streptomyces*. During his presentation in Philadelphia, Holland warned that the complexities of such treatments meant that only trained teams at major research centers should undertake such procedures. They were the ones best suited to administer the growing number of chemotherapy drugs.

Primum non nocere—that is Latin for "First do no harm." Although the origin of the phrase remains unclear, those words are often coupled with the doctor's Hippocratic oath, which pledges "to abstain from doing harm." Despite this guiding principle in medicine, Holland began to suggest that there may be exceptions to the rule.

"[It] goes back to an editorial I wrote for the *American Journal of Medicine* in 1966," he told me decades later. "In that piece, I wrote that if you treat everybody so nobody gets toxic, then you will have no effect on the tumor or the disease. Every study I've been involved with, you have to have some evidence of the drug's effect. We've yet to find a drug that has some effect on the tumor or whatever you're dealing with and has no effect on normal tissue."

In other words, some harm may be warranted to reach a desired result—or even a cure.

For raising this point, Holland said, "I have been criticized up, down, and sidewise by more conservative people in the medical community. Back in the beginning, when we were really getting started, Tom Frei and I were considered to be radical ragamuffins by many of them.

"Maybe we didn't play by the rules that others had. But we could point to remissions, which other people and their treatments didn't have, and more of our remissions soon became more long-lasting."

The notion of partial, and certainly complete, remissions would have been unthinkable a generation or so ago. Since the early days of modern medicine, the symptoms of leukemia—enlarged glands, fatigue, and bleeding—had been duly recorded, and they invariably led to death. One of the first documented cases of a child suffering from leukemia occurred more than a century before Holland's new doctrine. In 1860, in Germany, a five-year-old girl, remembered today as Maria, became exhausted, sleeping for extended periods of time. Red splotches appeared on her arms and legs and then her torso. A sample of her blood was examined under a microscope, a relatively new device to clinical medicine at the time. A few years before, in 1845, leukemia had first been diagnosed in an adult, and the patient's blood was found to be thick with "colorless globules or white blood cells." For Maria, the ailment was remarkably similar, and once again the illness proved to be sudden, mysterious, and fatal. Early treatments included leeches and arsenic, "which have been shown to be useless," according to a presentation about leukemia held at the Medical Society of London in the late 1800s.

Today, the American Cancer Society details that childhood leukemia is "often caused by problems in the child's bone marrow. . . . As leukemia cells build up in the marrow, they can crowd out the normal blood cell–making cells. As a result, a child may not have enough normal red blood cells, white blood cells, and blood platelets."

Leukemia is the most common form of cancer in children younger than fifteen years. A blood smear can reveal immature white blood cells, called lymphoblasts, that rapidly crowd out the healthy blood cells. (The word "leukemia" is derived from the Greek for "white blood.") Soon the system becomes so unbalanced that it can barely function. Patients suffering from leukemia not only bleed internally, with swelling of the liver and spleen, but they can bleed from the nose and ears too. The term "cancer," far from referring to a single disease, covers more than two hundred illnesses, with the common factor being the uncontrollable proliferation of malignant cells. That was the starting point for many of the pioneers in leukemia research—how to stop the acute growth of malignant cells.

Early in Holland's career, a colleague at the National Cancer Institute showed him how to isolate an enzyme from a pig's liver. Although the younger doctor explained the basic concepts, Holland did much of the work himself. There were few specialists or extra technicians to do such tasks back then. In those years, the leukemia doctors were usually on their own—free to develop their new theories and put in the necessary grunt work, too.

In isolating the enzyme, Holland began to envision how the growing number of chemotherapy drugs could target specific sites in DNA development. For example, 6-MP and methotrexate were shown to impact purine synthesis, a key process in cell construction. Daunomycin could target the cancer as the DNA strands were formed. Vincristine could influence the function of microtubules, the protein structures that help cells maintain their shape and assist in cell division.

That different chemotherapy drugs could be effective at different stages in the formation of DNA and cells "was very exciting and novel at the time," Holland said.

No matter where the cancer cells were discovered, most leukemia specialists soon agreed that the cancer cells had to be fully obliterated. Even if 99.99 percent of the cancer was eliminated, enough of it still remained to eventually cause a relapse.

"That's what we were up against," said Jerry Yates, who became Holland's chief associate at Roswell Park. "If you left the cancer any opening, any opening at all, it did the patient no good in the long run. Eventually, it would return. That's what the clinical trials showed time and time again. That the cancer would find a way to come back, perhaps stronger this time around. That's what kind of disease leukemia is."

Leukemia could be beaten, Holland told his peers, but only if the chemotherapy drugs were used in ever-changing combinations and delivered to the patient at the stages when the disease was at its most vulnerable. His aggressive approach in battling leukemia continued to draw criticism from many quarters. At a meeting of the American College of Physicians, with several thousand members in attendance, the gathering became a showdown between Holland and Dr. William Crosby, Jr., a leading hematologist at the Walter Reed Medical Center.

Crosby questioned Holland's methods, suggesting that they may be unethical. Holland recalled that Crosby implied that the new methods perhaps hastened the passing of those with leukemia. Holland rebutted Crosby's claims by presenting a woman who had gone into remission due to the new procedures that he championed.

In the medical journal *Blood*, Dr. William Dameshek and others cautioned that such procedures were "new ways with old drugs" and "are presently poorly understood." The article continued, "It is conceivable that in the enthusiasm for major, and even minor, remissions that can now be produced in acute leukemia by a variety of agents," they wrote, "perspective may be lost regarding this terrible disease."

Even Sidney Farber, acknowledged as the father of chemotherapy, recommended that the new cancer drugs be better tested— one at a time, when possible—instead of in an increasing number of combinations. Growing up in Buffalo, Farber had witnessed the 1918 flu epidemic, when the city lost nearly 3,000 residents. After graduating from Harvard Medical School, Farber began at Children's Hospital in Boston and had early success treating children with leukemia. In 1947, ten of the sixteen young patients he treated with a folic acid–blocking agent went into temporary remission. It marked the first time a drug tested as an anticancer agent proved effective against leukemia.

Despite such success, Farber was reluctant to push further, especially when it came to giving children high dosages of several chemotherapy drugs at the same time. "I will not injure two children to save one," he once told a colleague.

In many ways, the caution and skepticism were understandable. Several of the new chemotherapy drugs were derived from mustard gas. The possible benefits of the gas against cancer were first noticed during World War I and then rediscovered during World War II. Studies found that the gas decimated normal white blood cells, which led some in the medical world to wonder if similar measures could eliminate destructive leukemic cells in cancer. These potentially lethal combinations of new medicines were increasingly combined with blood transfusions.

Certainly this was progress, Holland, Pinkel, and the other so-called cancer cowboys agreed. But they also contended that too many patients were unnecessarily dying when every new procedure and every new drug was investigated as methodically as the medical establishment required.

"One could argue that we could have done a better job of convincing the medical community, our peers, of what we were doing," Yates said. "But at the time, in the 1960s and 1970s, we were much more focused on solving the problem itself, finding a cure. James Holland and others soon realized that we were on to something. That we were showing real results with our approach. If anything, we ended up taking a degree of pride in all the criticism we received. Let them call us what they want. We were going to push ahead anyway. If anything, the criticism, the name-calling brought us closer together."

The NCI began a worldwide search for more compounds that could be deployed as chemotherapy drugs. As Emil Freireich pointed out, NCI Director C. Gordon Zubrod was an expert in infectious diseases, and "they had learned that if you gave two drugs it was more effective." If that was the case, perhaps three or four or five would do an even better job.

Pinkel added, "When the children were in remission, they could be pretty healthy. But on average, youngsters with ALL would last about a year and a half at most when we used one drug at a time."

With some graduates from U.S. medical schools reluctant to join their ranks, Roswell Park and other research hospitals regularly turned to doctors from overseas. They arrived on two- or three-year fellowships, and one of them became my brother's favorite.

Abdul Khaliq, a proud Muslim, was the doctor in charge one day when my mother stepped off the elevator on the fifth floor at Roswell Park and was almost run over by Eric barreling down the corridor on a tricycle.

When Mom began to discipline Eric, the doctor stepped in.

"I don't want to hear any more about this," Khaliq said. "Around here, it's eye for an eye. Please remember that, dear woman."

After briefly detailing that morning's treatment, how Eric had endured a spinal tap and another round of chemotherapy, he invited my brother to punch him in the gut.

"Give me a good one," the doctor ordered, and Eric promptly did so.

As both of them broke into laughter, the doctor scooped my brother up with one arm and put him on his shoulders. Then the two of them, still laughing, went striding down the hallway, leaving my bewildered mother in their wake.

Due to the success of the chemotherapy regime, Eric was technically an outpatient at Roswell Park. Still, he needed to spend significant time at the hospital off Main Street in Buffalo. These visits sometimes meant an overnight or longer stay. Through it all, he reveled in telling stories about his other world—tales from the other side.

One of his favorites had to do with one of our dogs. We had many over the years, usually Irish setters or golden retrievers. They weren't well trained and often strayed too close to Canal Road that ran by our house. One morning, one of our dogs was hit by a passing car. Nobody was at home, and those in the car didn't know what to do. So they loaded the dog in their trunk and drove him to the veterinarian in Middleport. Once they got there, they explained to the staff what had happened, and everyone went out to the car.

"But when they opened the trunk, guess what?" Eric said, and here he would pause, drawing out the punch line like a seasoned comic. "The trunk door went up and our dog jumped out. The vet and the rest of them couldn't believe it. For you see, our dog was fine. He was only knocked out. He proved to be around for a long, long time."

11

The doctors at Roswell Park, St. Jude, and the National Cancer Institute (NCI) rarely saw the world, and certainly not their collective past, in terms of major breakthroughs or medical milestones.

"The approach was to put in the time and follow the science," Lucius Sinks said. "Any real discoveries come at the end of what seemed to be a series of everyday, even boring, stretches of weeks and months strung together. If you're only concerned about some aha moment, if you're just sitting there waiting for those and concerned about nothing else, they never seem to come."

So the leukemia doctors did their work, fashioned the next clinical trial, and wrote another set of protocols. In doing so, they were spiritual, in their own way. In ancient thought, there is always the light and the dark, the passive and aggressive, the yin and the yang. The world often stands astride these two opposing yet complementary forces. As Thu Nguyen, my Buddhist teacher, once told me, "Did you notice the dot? In the field of white, in that drawing, there is always a small dot of black and in the black field there is always a dot of white. Nothing is ever totally one thing or another."

For doctors searching for a cure to leukemia, this meant that even the most devastating piece of bad news could hold a glimmer of hope. Conversely, even a string of great trial results—what the rest of us would consider a breakthrough—didn't mean everything had been decided and settled. Undoubtedly, another dot of uncertainty would crop up.

Doctors had determined that the bone marrow didn't function properly in patients with leukemia. Because of this, the platelet level in the blood plummeted and normal white blood cells were not sufficiently produced. Without enough platelets, the patients often began to bleed. That could occur in the nose, as sometimes happened with my brother. As soon as the packing was removed, the bleeding would start again.

"Or the bleeding would start from the mouth or coughing up blood or a rash, a red rash on the skin typical of bleeding, would occur," Dr. Emil "Tom" Frei said. "Or massive bleeding into the skin or bleeding into the urine or the bowel or even the brain. And once it started, it would progressively get worse."

At the National Cancer Institute, the director, C. Gordon Zubrod, regularly accompanied his doctors on their rounds. One morning, they came upon a four-year-old child who was breathing irregularly because he was bleeding so much from the nose and mouth. As the doctors entered the room, they saw several nurses scrubbing the blood off the walls and once again changing the sheets.

Zubrod turned to Dr. Emil Freireich and asked him, "Why don't you do something about this bleeding?"

In examining the blood work for his leukemia patients, Freireich saw that they were severely lacking in platelets. He decided to act on what he saw as the cause-and-effect relationship between that condition and the bleeding. Platelets, or thrombocytes, are components that are essential in helping blood clot. In a healthy person, platelets come together to form plugs in blood vessel injuries.

That led the doctors to consider whether, if they could somehow give their patients more platelets, it would help stop the bleeding.

Freireich and Frei at the NCI and Holland at Roswell Park proposed new clinical trials regarding platelets. That's when they ran into their first stumbling block. And the opposition was in-house: the NCI blood bank wanted no part of any additional procedures.

At the time, the blood bank "was very devoted to the heart transplant, the heart surgery program, for which they needed a lot of blood," Frei recalled. "So they weren't too anxious to supply us with platelets unless there was some reason to think that they worked. And nobody thought that they worked. That is, the power structure didn't think that they worked."

Initially, the old guard refused to participate in any studies about platelets and how patients could be helped through blood transfusions. Matters came to a head during a divisive meeting at the NCI. Frei and Freireich and their supporters made their case, only to be rebuked by a senior hematologist. The meeting began to break up with both sides still in their respective corners when Zubrod took the floor.

"We may not cure leukemia today or tomorrow or ever," he told the group, "but if we're going to cure it, it's by incremental steps, by facing each obstacle as we go along. One obstacle is bleeding. One possible way of controlling that is with platelet transfusion and we have got to do that. I, as clinical director of the National Cancer Institute, am obligated to see that that's done." The leukemia doctors had been given their chance. Now they had to deliver.

Freireich took the lead on a new study in which some patients were randomly allocated a bottle of fresh blood from which the platelets had been removed and other patients were given a bottle of fresh blood that contained platelets. The results overwhelmingly demonstrated the importance of more platelets. Eighteen of the twenty patients who received the fresh blood with the platelets responded favorably. Few in the group receiving blood without additional platelets showed any improvement at all.

Still, the critics remained vocal. So platelets worked? What about the problem of infection? In the early 1960s, it was estimated that 50 percent of the children with leukemia were dying from infections. Despite the use of antibiotics, infections remained the leading cause of death for many patients.

"So what are we going to do about that?" Freireich said. "Well, we did the same thing we did with platelets."

Tests in the lab revealed that many of the kids didn't have enough granulocytes in their systems to travel to the site of an infection. These white blood cells have small granules or particles that contain proteins to bolster the immune system. At first, patients were given granulocytes from normal, healthy donors, but that approach was found to be "totally useless," Freireich said. Instead, the doctors began to take such infection-fighting agents from patients with chronic leukemia. Often their granulocyte concentrations were one hundred to two hundred times higher than normal.

"Oh, my God, if you tried doing that [today], they'd lock you up like you were insane . . . ," Freireich said decades later. "But in that day, in that age, Zubrod said, 'Sounds crazy. Let's do it.'"

That said, gathering enough blood that was rich in platelets and granulocytes was next to impossible in the 1960s. Although primitive blood separators were available, none of them could handle a job this large and complex. That's why the leukemia doctors decided to build their own "continuous flow centrifuge machine"— in other words, an apparatus that could separate out such valuable elements in an inexpensive and timely fashion.

At first, Freireich tried to do it on his own, with plastic tubes soon running all over his lab at the NCI. He wasn't making much progress when a guy named George Judson knocked on his door one morning. Judson's ten-year-old son suffered from leukemia. Frei remembered that the Judson family didn't have much money, but the father worked at IBM as a developmental engineer. And the father wanted to help in any way he could.

Freireich told him about this pipe dream for a centrifuge machine, a blood cell apparatus to better separate blood. Judson listened, and in a few months he returned, saying he had been given a paid leave from his job at IBM. He was ready to commute down from his home in central New York and build this new machine. With him, Judson brought along several pieces of heavy hardware, plastic, screws, and bolts.

"All of us helped with it," Frei said, "but Jay and this engineer were there for the most part. We actually saw it develop in the room."

Freireich said that Judson "would pirate junk parts out of the factories. . . . We took this Mickey Mouse claptrap thing and we collected white cells from patients with chronic granulocytic leukemia who were being donors for our granulocytes. We showed it would work. But everything was claptrap, you know. The pumps didn't work well, the seals were breaking. So the idea was correct, but we didn't have the equipment."

Once again, Zubrod intervened, convincing an advisory committee to pony up several thousand dollars, and soon a contract was issued for the machine's further development. Following Freireich and Judson's semblance of a blueprint, the first continuous-flow blood cell separator was constructed and soon made available to hospitals.

Roswell Park was named by the NCI to test the blood cell machine. The hospital's new donor center, one of the first in the country, was established by Dr. Elias Cohen, and between 1964 and 1978, the deaths due to excessive bleeding fell from 60 to 15 percent as the platelet-heightened blood made it easier for patients' blood to clot.

With the donor system up and going, now augmented by the IBM blood cell machine 2990 and later by the IBM 2991, the leukemia doctors made a new rule for their daily rounds. "If anyone ever saw a drop of blood in the room," Freireich said, "then the doctor was immediately reprimanded because we knew how to control it. And there was no blood on the walls, no blood on the bedsheets. And that's true today. If you go in[to] a leukemia ward, you won't see anybody bleeding."

12

In October 1967, Eric relapsed and was pulled from Study No. 6608. A month before, he had begun kindergarten at Gasport Elementary, a ten-minute bus ride down Route 31 from our home on Canal Road. On a summary sheet from Roswell Park, it was noted in the right-hand margin that his tonsils were red and enlarged. In addition, a reading of Eric's bone marrow showed an increase in white blood cells. Another round of vincristine and prednisone was ordered. This combination would become the fallback for my brother's treatment. Once again, the one-two punch did the trick, and Eric technically went into remission. A week before Thanksgiving, he was shifted to biweekly treatments of methotrexate. These sometimes required an overnight stay at Roswell Park.

By now, my parents had learned what the doctors were well aware of: cancer remains a disease of mutations and often uncontrollable growth. Believe you have it pinned down, finally trapped in a corner, and it will adapt and recover and grow faster than any normal cell. Finding a cure for all the different strands and variations that are cancer can border on the absurd. Yet the leukemia doctors embraced the riddle, even the impossibility of this task. What others deemed hopeless, they decided was well worth the effort. Where others demanded some kind of pattern, cadence, or logic, they accepted how irrational all of it could be. They soon learned that nothing stayed the same day to day, and certainly not month to month or year to year, with childhood leukemia. To take it on, one needed to be as mindful, as centered in the moment, as the disease itself seemed to be. In a way, we began to practice the same approach as a family.

Out on the water, as we ventured farther and farther from the south shore of Lake Ontario, we were reminded how fast the world could change. Susan, for example, remembered the afternoon we were blindsided by a squall line. This was well before weather radar and cell phones and other such warnings. The only way to know that a squall line was heading toward us was to keep a keen eye on the horizon and listen for lightning-induced crackles on the AM radio.

Squall lines form ahead of a cold front and sustain themselves by producing a strong updraft. They can be accompanied by gusting winds, lightning, hail, and sometimes consist of several thunderstorms banded together in a dark line.

On this day, Susan went to the foredeck to drop the jib. Dad told her to put on a life jacket and harness before leaving the safety of the cockpit, and to clip into the lifelines running along the sides of the boat as she made her way forward, past the mast. Susan gave him a curious look, almost questioning his order. After all, right above us it was a beautiful sunny day. But then Dad nodded to a dark line of clouds on the western horizon, well out over the lake. They had flattened tops and dark underbellies, a sure sign of heavy weather. Beneath the approaching bank of clouds, barely visible to the naked eye, the blue water had given way to black seas, already dotted with white caps.

In short order, the rest of us had reefed the mainsail and attached jumper cables to the metal stays running down from the mast. This was a last resort—an attempt to direct any lightning hits into the water instead of through the boat.

My sister quickly dropped the jib. Yet she couldn't resist lingering on the foredeck for a better look at the approaching weather. Soon the squall line hit us with such ferocity that the boat rolled briefly over on its side, even though we flew so little sail. Susan kept her footing and hung on to the lifelines. From the cockpit, I saw her open her mouth. Almost blinded by the storm, she squinted into the direction of the squall line and shook her head.

For a moment or two, the wind moaned through the metal rigging and rocked our boat from side to side. We heard the crack of thunder, and on both sides, the sky filled with lightning. Then, almost as soon as it had come on us, the squall line moved on. Soaked to the bone, Susan returned to the cockpit, and Chris ducked below to fetch her a towel.

"What were you doing up there?" I whispered, not wanting to get her in trouble with Dad.

"Singing," she said

"Singing? But why?"

"It made me laugh," she grinned. "How the wind swept away the words away from me before I could even hear them."

I looked at her as if she was crazy. My sister never ceased to amaze me. Yet in the months ahead, I began to understand her tenacity and gallows humor in such conditions. Perhaps she realized that the squall line was somehow an omen for what we would encounter, on and off the water. Sometimes such storms would be on us before we knew it, and the only thing we could do was to hang on and find the courage to sing through it all.

"ARE YOU MAKING PROGRESS?" Lucius Sinks asked.

We were back at our table at the Boar's Head, the official hotel of the University of Virginia in Charlottesville. The table for two overlooked the vast grounds and the Blue Ridge Mountains to the west. After several months of trying to understand leukemia and all its ramifications, I had turned to Sinks again for help.

"I'm getting there," I said. "But all of the drugs my brother was on—methotrexate, 6-MP, cyclophosphamide, daunomycin—they all get jumbled up on my end."

Sinks nodded.

"They can act very differently," he said. "Take prednisone, for example. As you know, it is a steroid and found to be generally effective against leukemia. For some reason, it becomes even more effective when you pair it with vincristine. Why? Nobody is exactly sure. We certainly didn't know precisely back then. Perhaps they do now, but that doesn't really matter."

"Why not?"

Sinks paused, gathering his thoughts. "What you have to keep in mind is that our work with these drugs, especially early on, was guesswork," he said.

"Guesswork?"

"We wanted to find the ones that were effective at a particular time, in a particular situation," Sinks continued. "That's what the clinical trials were all about. Exactly why one particular drug worked and another one that we tried didn't was sometimes a secondary concern. Our focus was always on the patients. What could work against this disease right now? As I've told you, the focus was on the day to day, the specifics in terms of what worked for the patient."

I nodded, trying to make sense of this. "I feel like I'm lost in the tall grass with all the terminology," I told him.

"There's a lot there. But remember that with each patient, there's a particular order of treatment. One drug is tried and another, perhaps now in combination like prednisone and vincristine. In all likelihood, the patient becomes part of a clinical trial, and then

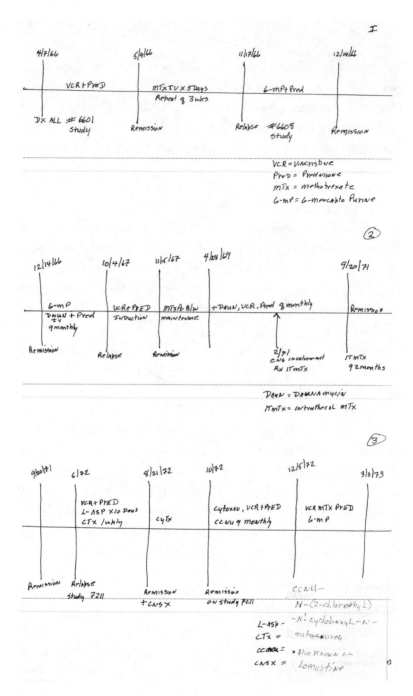

Hand-drawn chart by Dr. Lucius Sinks. Eric Wendel's chemotherapy drugs from April 7, 1966, to March 3, 1973, Roswell Park. Vertical lines indicate relapse or remission.

something else is tried when the previous drug or combination isn't found to be effective anymore. It is one step and then another and another. I'd like to say it was all planned out, but it never was. We were going step by step too, trying one thing and then another, moving as fast as we could. Find that path with your brother. That can help you better understand it all much better."

A week later, a manila envelope arrived in the mail from Sinks. At one of our previous meetings, I had given him what I had of Eric's medical records. Despite huge gaps in the information, Sinks had been able to put together a three-page chart detailing all my brother's medicines and treatments.

I spread the pages out on my desk, seeing the progression for the first time. How those first dosages of vincristine and prednisone in spring 1966 led to the methotrexate via IV and then to the 6-MP and prednisone, and so forth and so on. Sinks brought this all together to form one horizontal line, moving left to right across the page, with vertical lines marking the times when Eric technically fell into remission or relapsed.

I gazed on the pages and began to understand how it could all fit together.

13

By Eric's third year at Roswell Park, he had been on five different chemotherapy drugs in a half-dozen different combinations. About the only consistency displayed in Sinks's flowchart was the one-two punch of prednisone and vincristine, which was prescribed when my brother relapsed or really struggled.

When his condition stabilized, Eric next participated in a maintenance program of biweekly doses of methotrexate, the chemotherapy drug that could inhibit DNA synthesis at several key stages and that was used in multiple ways in chemotherapy. In addition to being taken in pill form, methotrexate had found a new role in intrathecal therapy. That meant injecting the drug directly into the spinal canal, into the subarachnoid space that reaches the cerebrospinal fluid surrounding the spinal cord on up to the brain itself. Eventually, this would become a key alternative to the more harmful use of radiation.

Today, moving onto a maintenance program can be viewed as being one step away from being cured. Yet in the late 1960s, despite the growing number of chemotherapy drugs, the path to long-term remission was far from certain. Doctors were making progress, especially with the spinal canal infusion. But nobody dared talk about a cure. Eric knew as well as anybody that any medical procedure remained another roll of the dice.

One afternoon Eric was with Mom in the play area in the 5 East Unit, the children's floor at Roswell Park. The two of them were working on a jigsaw puzzle at the big table close to the window. The pieces of another puzzle—a pastoral landscape or a famous city—were usually scattered across the tabletop, and anybody could try their hand when they had a moment.

On this afternoon, one of the younger doctors stopped by to talk with my mother.

"So you like puzzles?" he asked Eric.

My brother hadn't really been paying attention to their conversation. Sometimes such talk was too nice, too contrived for him. But he looked up at the doctor and replied, "I hope you like puzzles too. I hope you're real good at them."

Left unspoken was that so much of what was going on at Roswell Park resembled a complex, exhausting puzzle, with an ever-increasing number of variables. When best to roll out the 6-MP or daunomycin? And in what dosage? Too small an amount would hardly put a dent in the cancer. Too much could harm, even kill a patient. Even prednisone, an old standby, caused some patients to become delirious. Others suffered from a burning sensation in the fingers and feet. Due to VAMP and other groundbreaking clinical trials, it had been determined that a four-drug regimen often worked better than a three-drug "cocktail" and usually better than two drugs. And soon more cancer-fighting drugs would become available—cyclophosphamide, lomustine, and Cytoxan. So much depended on how fast the doctors could put the pieces together.

Elsewhere in 1968, there were puzzles aplenty. It ranked among the most tumultuous years in the nation's history. The Vietnam War, which spiked with the Tet Offensive, soon divided the nation.

Then Dr. Martin Luther King and Bobby Kennedy were assassinated. Still, at Roswell Park, my parents continued to receive mostly good news.

"ALL in complete remission," began one update. "This healthy-looking boy returns for follow-up as scheduled."

"He is asymptomatic except for a mild cough without production of sputum," was the documentation for the next visit.

Eric's visits to Buffalo became more regular as the maintenance regiment of methotrexate (20 milligrams twice weekly) continued to keep the leukemia at bay. Eric's only complaints were occasional sores in his mouth, and the doctors noticed a slight lack of tendon reflexes in both legs. Obesity, muscle and tendon weakness, and long-term cardiac disease were a few of the adverse effects of cancer treatment at the time. That said, the doctors decided that Eric was healthy enough to receive a measles vaccine and polio vaccine a few weeks later. At the time, there was no vaccine for chicken pox.

MY MOTHER GREW up outside of Flint, Michigan, and her father, Gordon Harry, had worked as an engineer for General Motors. When he retired, he and his wife, Mimi, moved into a two-bedroom cottage with lakefront access. Grandpa Gord soon bought another small cottage two lots down on Lake Leelanau, and that's where we stayed when we visited for a few weeks every summer.

Up in Michigan, the beach and grounds were our grandfather's domain. He erected two barge-like jetties that extended 20 feet into the lake, funneling sand onto the beach. When we were there, Grandpa Gord rose at dawn, raking the beach in preparation for another day's activity. Then he came up the stairs from the water, across the small lawn, and into the kitchen, where he daily prepared "a lumberman's breakfast" for his guests.

Growing up I became closer to my other grandfather, Leon, who lived a few miles away from us in Lockport. And perhaps such things are ordained early on. My middle name was Lee, after my Grandpa Leon, or Lee, as he liked to be called. Eric's middle name was Gordon, and the two of them resembled each other—lighter hair and fairer skin, a full face, and a smile that had to be earned.

Putting together a lumberman's breakfast took time. "This isn't a quick-order place," he once reminded me.

As Gord cooked the bacon and scrambled the eggs and began to flip the pancakes, we kids gathered in the "crud room," which was a cubbyhole of a place just off the gravel driveway. We were a hungry lot at that hour. Occasionally, our cousins from California would overlap with our time in town, and all nine of us would come together, as surly and as sullen as any backwater saloon crowd west of the Pecos.

To try to keep us quiet until the adults arose and the full breakfast could be served, Grandpa Gord set out Kellogg's variety packs of cereal, milk, bowls, and plastic spoons on the picnic table where we gathered. The most coveted brands in the variety packs were Sugar Pops, Fruit Loops, and Frosted Flakes—all the fine-grade sugary stuff.

One morning when our cousins were in town, a raging argument broke out about who should have the next pick of cereal. That prompted Eric to find Grandpa Gord in the kitchen.

"They're going to tear each other apart," he grimly told his namesake. "Where's the dice?"

When you stayed at my grandfather's house in Michigan, matters of import, great and small, were settled with a roll of the dice. The two pieces came in a leather cup, like you would find at a bar, and if a real argument flared up, one shook the dice and rolled them out. High score won. No questions asked.

Usually, the dice were kept on a shelf in the crud room. But on this morning, with a new variety pack of cereal ready to be consumed, the cup had gone missing. None of us had thought to look for it, except for Eric.

"Here you go," Gord told him. "It ended up in here somehow."

Had the adults resorted to gambling and drinking games after we kids had fallen asleep? I never got to the bottom of that one. But Eric took the leather cup and returned to the crud room, quelling the uprising. A roll of the dice seemed somehow equitable to everyone—something we could all agree on.

14

James Holland became a doctor thanks to what he calls "a series of fortunate mistakes." The son of a prominent lawyer in Morristown, New Jersey, Holland was raised to go into law too. But that changed when he took a course in biology at Princeton University and became enthralled with seeing cells under a microscope.

"I was just captivated by what I saw," he said. "Sometimes life works like that. Things suddenly turn and you're off and heading in a totally different direction."

During the Korean War, Holland was in the U.S. Army and had secured an entry position at Columbia-Presbyterian University, only to have President Harry Truman extend the military service time. When Columbia couldn't hold the position for him, Holland later went to Francis Delafield Hospital, also in New York City, which had opened to care for cancer patients. Holland's plan was to mark time at Delafield until a new slot became available at Columbia. Yet Holland soon became intrigued with cancer and how best to manage it.

Early on at Delafield, he treated a baby girl named Josephine who was suffering from leukemia. He used aminopterin, now recognized as the first chemotherapeutic agent for acute leukemia in children, and the four-year-old regained her health. The turnaround was so startling that other doctors wanted to see for themselves, and a viewing was arranged in the semicircular amphitheater at Presbyterian Hospital. On the day of the event, Holland brought in brightly colored balloons and fastened them to the brass railings that cordoned off the area in an effort to reassure his young patient. When the crowd of doctors arrived, Josephine was smiling, captivated by the balloons, and the visit went off without hitch.

Unfortunately, Josephine soon relapsed, and then she again had "the anguish of dealing with nosebleeds, gum bleeding and bruises in the skin; and primitive antibiotics were all we had available then to treat infections," he later told Dr. John Laszlo. "And she was only a child, a crying child." Holland added, "There was just unbelievable trauma for everybody concerned. I was only a resident at the time, and this was my first case of leukemia after I had come back from the army, and the first cancer patient that I put into remission."

Soon Columbia called, saying that a position had opened up there. But Holland turned them down. He had found his place in medicine: it was being a cancer doctor.

"Deep down just about everybody likes mysteries and I don't believe there's anything better in the world than solving them," he said. "You look at cancer and realize how much we don't know and then you realize how much still needs to be done. It's an opportunity for young, vigorous people—a chance for them to say they want to be a part of that. Something so much bigger than themselves.

"The people I was surrounded by back then, that I'm still surrounded by today, we like to make discoveries. That's what keeps us going. In a way, I feel sorry for people in other fields. They're often looking at things that are pretty matter-of-fact. Early in my career, I realized that in dealing with cancer, that we were looking at the bigger picture. Issues like what makes one cell stay alive and what makes another cell die? That's important, challenging work, I think. It's what has kept me going through the years."

Holland was soon called to the National Cancer Institute, where he worked with Lloyd Law, one of the first doctors to use cancer drugs in combinations. With Law's help, Holland began testing a combination of 6-MP and methotrexate, which proved successful in the early years of leukemia research.

Holland arrived at Roswell Park late in 1954, brought aboard by George Moore, the energetic new director. Moore was determined to hire young, dynamic physicians to head the various departments at his growing hospital complex. Even though Holland wasn't thirty years old yet, he was appointed as one of three chiefs of medicine for the expanding cancer research facility. With the move, Holland saw his salary jump from $7,600 to $11,300 a year. He soon married Jimmie Holland, who would become a key player in the growing field of psycho-oncology, where psychology and oncology came together for cancer treatment.

Many consider this to be the beginning of a golden era at Roswell Park. Holland's contemporaries included Donald Pinkel, who was beginning to calculate more effective drug dosages for children with leukemia. Dr. Joseph Sokal and his staff developed new protocols for chemotherapy, and Dr. Avery Sandberg investigated the role of chromosomes in causing cancer. There were plenty of egos in play, and Holland recalled that he and Moore "used to fight like cats and dogs. But we always respected each other."

Dr. Edwin Mirand, the author of *Legacy and History of Roswell Park Cancer Institute*, acknowledges that "the interaction between the clinicians and scientists was intense." Yet he adds that many of

Moore's hires soon became known far beyond the confines of Roswell Park "for the quality and creativity of their work."

Back at the NCI, Gordon Zubrod asked Holland if he would continue to be involved in the leukemia program even though he was now in Buffalo. Holland agreed and decided to augment the study of 6-MP and methotrexate at Roswell Park. Emil "Tom" Frei at the NCI took over many of the administrative chores for the collaborative effort and was soon joined by Emil Freireich at the NCI and Pinkel in Buffalo. In the beginning, Pinkel said, it "was basically us four."

That was the inception of the Acute Leukemia Group B (ALGB), which would later be renamed the Cancer and Leukemia Group B, or CALGB. Members of the cancer research cooperative began to meet every other month, going over initial results and standardizing forms and clinical trial criteria. The Walter Reed Medical Center, the Medical College of Virginia, and the University of Maryland were among the other institutions that soon joined the effort.

Early on, the ALGB struggled to find enough children with leukemia to participate in its new studies. Too many family doctors viewed ALGB with deep suspicion. After all, cancer, especially in kids, was often considered to be incurable. Why put them through the ordeal of combination drug therapy, blood work, and the like?

"So we had to recruit patients," Freireich said. "So what we did is systematically begin to visit medical societies, hospitals, clinics, patient advocate groups, and we advertised what we were doing. Here's the research we're doing. Trying to impress them with our compassion.

"We don't experiment, we give them treatment, we were making progress. We began to build a practice. And that was item number one—we had to build a practice. We had to be good. We had to have good relations with parents, with children, and universities."

The ability to motivate people with words soon became one of Holland's chief assets. In 1965, he published an article entitled "Obstacles to the Control of Acute Leukemia" in the *CA: Cancer Journal for Clinicians.* Much of it had been originally presented at a symposium sponsored by the American Cancer Society and the National Cancer Institute. The peer-reviewed publication was the most widely circulated oncology journal at the time, going out to more than 100,000 readers and professionals. In the five-page piece, Holland cited the success that the combination of vincristine and prednisone had had against cancer. Yet what got the medical world buzzing was the confidence, the sheer chutzpah, that Holland exhibited in his belief that childhood leukemia could be conquered in the years ahead   perhaps as early as the next decade. Despite the pessimism in many quarters, Holland insisted "that nearly every obstacle appears to be identifiable and approachable—if not surmountable—at present or in the immediate future." Holland added that the "data, result, and concepts are now such as to allow legitimate informed discussion, planning, and execution of attempts to cure acute leukemia rather than merely palliate it. . . . It is in times of universal challenge accepted by every man that giant strides are made."

Jerry Yates was practicing medicine in California when he read Holland's article. His initial reaction? "I need to talk to this man. I need to find a way to work for him."

Yates had recently treated a patient who had died of testicular cancer. The man was twenty-seven years old, about the same age as Yates at the time. The young doctor was devastated by his patient's passing. A few weeks later, Yates came upon Holland's article.

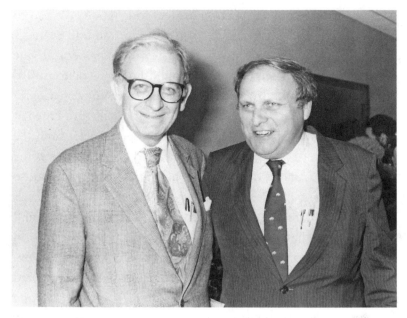

Dr. James Holland (left) and Dr. Jerome Yates. Courtesy of Dr. Jerome Yates.

"And it just rocked me. It just snapped me out of this state I was in," Yates said. "James Holland was so far ahead of the rest of us. He saw a different world out there—one of real possibility. One in which people could be, did we dare say it, cured? To hear something like that, when you're working in many of the same areas of care . . . well, it meant everything to me at the time."

Yates landed an interview at Roswell Park and spent much of the day with Holland, going on rounds, talking about the growing possibilities in terms of leukemia care. Their conversation carried on into the late afternoon as Holland drove Yates to the Buffalo airport. When the official job offer arrived from Roswell Park, Yates quickly accepted. He did so even though Holland had warned him about the long hours, the hard winters in western New York, and the often devastating clinical trial results.

"When I look back on those days, it was a good thing that we had to do many of the initial tests ourselves," Yates said. "There was no sending the patient down the hall to an expert in this field or that. We had to be or become the experts. We had to be the first to learn many of the procedures, setting up the next clinical trial and its parameters. We had to do it because so much of the medicine was that new to everyone involved."

Nurse Audrey Tuttolomondo, who worked for two decades at Roswell Park, remembered Holland as a commanding presence. "A lot of it has to do with his voice," she said. "It turned heads and it demanded respect. It's this deep baritone-bass voice that could be heard from a long ways down any hallway."

Although Holland proved to be adept at empire building, the gatherings of the ALGB were regularly contentious, with the floor open to about anyone. Once a young doctor from the National Cancer Institute questioned the high dosages of methotrexate and cyclophosphamide the doctors were beginning to prescribe.

"My God, those doses are so dangerous," Holland remembered him saying. "You're going to kill children."

As a result, the ALGB cut the dosages of methotrexate for many of its patients from 15 milligrams per square meter of body surface to 12 milligrams per square meter and trimmed the cyclophosphamide almost in half. Eventually, the doctors with the ALGB determined that the higher doses of methotrexate indeed worked best in this case, especially when coupled with cyclophosphamide to briefly suppress the immune system.

"We got more information out of the study by these circuitous, serendipitous excursions than we would have by using the original plan," Holland said. "That said, we were always conscious of the time. We didn't have the luxury of it with most of our patients."

Holland remained the ALGB chairman for eighteen years, staying on even after a horse he was riding with his four-year-old daughter reared up and fell backward on top of him. Holland was able to throw his daughter clear (she was unharmed), but the horse crushed his pelvis. Holland soon made a full recovery.

Growing up, Holland had been taught poetry by his father, and he found motivation and solace in the power of words. I once asked him if he would recite a few lines from a poem, perhaps a favorite of his. "How did you know that about me?" Holland demanded. "That I learned poetry growing up?"

I told him that several of his friends and peers admired this quality about him.

"All right then," he replied. "How about a few lines from 'Elegy Written in a Country Churchyard.' You know it?"

I didn't.

"Well, you should. It's one of my favorites. You can look up the particulars about it." (Indeed, I found that the poem was written by Thomas Gray and was published in 1751. It runs 144 lines, and scholars believe it was inspired by the death of Richard West, Gray's friend and a fellow poet.)

Holland began in a voice that still holds one's undivided attention.

Full many a gem of purest ray serene,
The dark unfathom'd caves of ocean bear,
Full many a flow'r is born to blush unseen,
And waste its sweetness on the desert air.

"I love the cadence of that, how it rolls off the tongue," Holland said after reciting those lines. "I learned it when I was young and I've never forgotten it. To me, it's about believing good work can be done. How good work can be accomplished, if you're willing to push on."

Throughout the 1960s, Holland and the other doctors with the ALGB pushed on with the clinical trials—the documented reports of their efforts. Similar practices had proven effective earlier in the efforts against tuberculosis. The germs that cause tuberculosis were considered to be similar to cancer cells in that they soon become resistant to one drug or antibiotic. As a result, Holland, Pinkel, and others advocated a similar approach with the growing number of cancer drugs at their disposal.

Under Holland's supervision, with the National Cancer Institute's blessing, some groups of patients were treated in conventional ways and others received more radical procedures. None of the patients was told what he or she was being given. This was termed "masking," and doctors said it was crucial to the success of any trial.

In these early trials, some patients received chemotherapy drugs in combination, for example methotrexate and 6-MP. Others received just one drug and others a placebo. A pattern soon emerged that many agreed was indisputable: the more aggressive the treatment, the better the patients, especially young children, usually responded.

Decades later Holland maintained that those trials, "going back to the early ones, like 6601, were pivotal for us. They gave us a much quicker insight into what we were up against and what could be done."

Dr. Larry Norton at Memorial Sloan Kettering Cancer Center in New York said that such clinical trials at Roswell Park and elsewhere in the 1960s were "the most significant advance" in the campaign against cancer. "Innovative scientific ideas come along frequently," he added, "but they still have to be tested. Not everything logical is true, but everything that is true should be confirmed. And the major leap forward in the confirmation process was the emergence of the randomized controlled prospective trials."

Jerry Yates added, "The clinical trials were key because they helped us accelerate the treatment, really start to help our patients. By working cooperatively, we soon developed the methodology for looking at the clinical trial proceedings to see what was truly working. That is one of the big events that came out of the early treatment of cancer. We got a lot of criticism for it. But as Jim Holland would say, 'We have the documentation to show we're making progress.'"

That said, the leukemia doctors knew that too much chemotherapy, too many drugs in the system, could result in liver damage, sterility, and secondary episodes of cancer for the kids. So it was with some trepidation that the VAMP clinical trial combining vincristine, amethopterin (methotrexate), mercaptopurine (6-MP), and prednisone went ahead in 1961. The children in this protocol soon became very sick as the near-lethal combinations ravaged their systems. Some needed to be hooked up to respirators, while others nearly fell into a coma. Yet the examinations of those who pulled through revealed that their bone marrow was free of leukemia cells.

Another round of VAMP trials was completed, and the results indicated this particular combination of drugs had proven effective against cancer. As dosages were adjusted, more children moved into remission, and even critics had to admit that the leukemia doctors might be onto something.

In September 1963, however, several survivors of the VAMP clinical trials began to complain of headaches and tingling in the limbs. Even though subsequent bone marrow biopsies came back clean, tests of the kids' spinal fluid revealed that the cancer had found refuge in areas of the spinal cord and brain.

"This is because of the blood–brain barrier," Donald Pinkel said. "It's an old system in the body that helps keep poisons out of the brain. It's a good system. But it can also keep the chemo drugs out too. That created a sanctuary for the cancer and once it finds a safe haven, somewhere that the chemotherapy cannot reach, it can grow and grow and grow. We soon realized that we had to find a different way."

15

When Donald Pinkel returned home to Buffalo, becoming the head of pediatrics, he expected to be at Roswell Park "for the rest of my life." Yet when the winter of 1961 arrived, he developed a bad case of pneumonia that he couldn't shake. "Don, you have to get out of this climate," Pinkel's doctor told him. "Your lungs just won't clear up."

Reluctantly, the thirty-four-year-old Pinkel accepted an interview for a new job in Colorado. He was ready to visit there when officials at the proposed St. Jude Research Hospital in Memphis reached out to him. Danny Thomas was the driving force behind the new facility in western Tennessee. The actor had vowed to build a shrine to St. Jude Thaddeus if his career ever took wings: his personal deal with God. Once Thomas became a household name in the popular television show *Make Room for Daddy,* he discussed his plan with Catholic priest Samuel Stritch, a close friend and the archbishop of Chicago. Stritch told the actor that there were plenty of shrines. What was needed was another place to heal the sick.

After discussions about building such a hospital in Boston or St. Louis, Thomas decided "to put it in the South," said his daughter, Marlo Thomas, "and then Cardinal Stritch in Chicago said, 'I'll help you to put it in Memphis' because that's where he's from."

On the way to Colorado, Pinkel stopped off at Memphis, where he didn't mince words. He asked the hospital board and members of the University of Tennessee Medical School if they would "accept all children, including black children, at this hospital, and [would] there be complete integration in all levels—staff, nurses, everything?"

There was an awkward silence until one of the university chairmen spoke up. He freely used the N-word and told Pinkel that a few black patients would be fine—as long as the hospital wasn't overrun by patients of color.

Pinkel didn't say a word, but inside he recalled, "I boiled, boiled, boiled. I thought, 'Wow! That guy is giving me a challenge. To say I can't do that.'"

Pinkel's worst fears of the South had been borne out. After all, he had grown up in a large, liberal family in Buffalo, where a portrait of Abraham Lincoln hung on the wall. His ancestors had fought for the Union in the Civil War, and one of his great-uncles had been killed in the conflict. Personally, he vowed to never work in the South because "there was so much prejudice down there."

Pinkel visited Colorado, where he was offered "a sweetheart job." The university there already sported a state-of-the-art hospital on campus, with a quality staff and excellent students. It seemed to be an easy choice. Yet what nagged at Pinkel was that he had been challenged in Memphis. Back in high school, a coach had warned Pinkel that you "never run away from a fight. It'll be more and more difficult the further you run to fight back."

The next morning, Pinkel awoke and decided he would take the job in Memphis, building a hospital for Danny Thomas. Several of his closest friends were stunned. His mentor, Mitchell Rubin, who was from South Carolina, wrote Pinkel a long letter telling him, "You can't do that." But Pinkel's mind was made up.

He reached out to Edward Barry, the chairman of the board for the new hospital, and to Michael Tamer, the executive director for the American Lebanese Syrian Associated Charities. (Danny Thomas was Lebanese American.) If they weren't in his corner, Pinkel knew he had little chance of success in western Tennessee. The three met at a neutral site—a hotel room at the Conrad Hilton in Chicago. There Pinkel outlined his vision for the research hospital. How they would take care of all kinds of children, with the primary focus being on kids with cancer and other supposed incurable diseases, such as muscular dystrophy. Barry, like Pinkel, was Jesuit-educated and one of the most influential men in Memphis. The two of them soon hit it off.

"Our minds just met," Pinkel said. "It clicked. We didn't have to explain things. We were from the same background."

In comparison, Tamer hadn't finished high school, but he too believed strongly in everyone being on equal footing. He urged Pinkel and Barry to sort out the details, and he would focus on the big picture. At the end of the day, the three shook hands, and Pinkel officially took the job. A few weeks later, the doctor arrived in Memphis on the feast of St. Jude, which he took as a good omen.

"My mother had a devotion to St. Jude," Pinkel said. "She used to go down to Saint John Maron Church in Buffalo . . . to see a Father Shemalie, who was a typical Eastern Church holy man. She would bring donations and she asked him to pray for us.

"I remember when I took a scholarship exam for high school and everybody was hoping for a full scholarship. She called up Father Shemalie and said, 'Pray for my boy. He's taking a scholarship exam.' He said, 'I'll pray for him,' and he did. And when I got it, my mother said, 'Father Shemalie came through. St. Jude did it.'"

Pinkel remembered that his mother had a holy card with a special prayer to St. Jude, the patron of hope and impossible causes. She urged him to say that prayer every night.

That said, if Pinkel had known what awaited him in Memphis, he would have thought twice about taking the post. By the time he arrived, the new hospital was already running out of money, and he had to first become a fund-raiser to assure that the patient wing was even built.

Decades later, looking back on the move to Memphis, Pinkel said the job "was a very iffy proposition. But it sure got my attention. The people there told me they would support me, so I decided to find out."

The new doctor in town soon became involved with the African American community. When several local civil rights leaders were jailed and went on a hunger strike, Pinkel visited them and brought along infant formula. He told them to drink it to keep up their strength.

By the end of his first year, Pinkel had 126 patients at St. Jude. They were "girls and boys, black and white, Catholic, Protestant, and Jewish," as *Memphis* magazine later detailed. Just as important, Pinkel had assembled a medical staff of one hundred, many of whom took some cajoling to move to the South.

Despite early success, Pinkel realized that if he didn't fix a major problem with the local blood banks, little of the cancer research he was proposing would ever get off the ground. At the time, there was a steep markup from the donor level to the local hospitals in the Memphis area. Pinkel's new hospital was sometimes being charged as much as $35 a unit. So he appealed to the commanders at the nearby Millington Naval Air Station, urging the naval personnel and marines there to become regular blood donors. A system was worked out in which men in uniform received weekend passes to

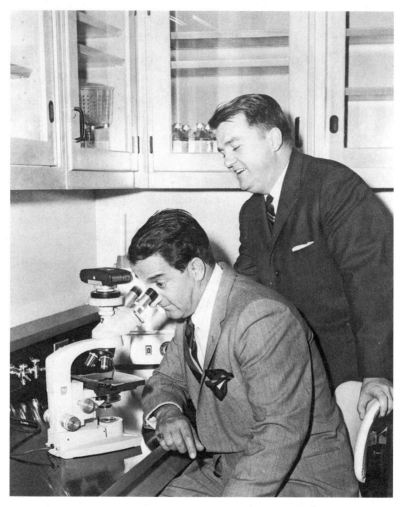

Danny Thomas (seated) and Dr. Donald Pinkel. Courtesy of St. Jude Children's Research Hospital.

Memphis for every blood donation they gave. Pinkel also recruited local college students and inmates at local prisons. In doing so, he formed a volunteer donor system in western Tennessee and, as he said years later, "broke the back of the local blood banks."

It was another step on a long road for Pinkel, where attitude was as important as anything for the doctor.

"As I've said, a sense of hopelessness pervaded the entire field— to the point that many in the medical community thought, 'Why bother to take on leukemia?'" he said decades later. "Nothing appeared like it was going to change, ever, and those of us battling to do something different? Well, lots of people thought we were nuts. And when you look back at what we had to overcome, not only in Memphis, but at other hospitals, like at Roswell Park, perhaps we were crazy. Maybe we had to be."

16

On this Friday morning, I was the first to arrive at what had become our regular table at the Boar's Head Inn. I liked getting here a little bit early, rehearsing in my mind what I needed to ask Lucius Sinks this time. Out the window, the sun had begun to break through the late-morning clouds on this day in early summer.

The room slowly filled with people, and the doctor appeared across the room. He was dressed in a polo shirt and khakis, with his cane in hand. In his opposite hand, he carried a large canvas bag. He broke into a smile as he approached our table.

"I brought you some homework," he said, placing the bag down with a thud between the place settings. "Go ahead, take a look."

I reached inside and pulled out a regular-size book with a blue cover. It was entitled *Conflicts in Childhood Cancer*. Sinks and another doctor were the coauthors.

"You can hang onto that one," Sinks said. "The other tome I'll need back at some point."

And a tome it was. So cumbersome that I struggled with both hands to lift the heavy book from the bag. *Cancer Medicine* 2nd ed., was the title of this one, and it had two authors, James F. Holland and Emil Frei III. With a reddish hardcover, it topped out at a whopping 2,465 pages.

Sinks chuckled at the look on my face. "I don't expect you to read it all," he said as we sat down, the two books lying in the middle of the table between us. "But with the questions you're asking, you might as well go right to the source material. When it comes to the science of leukemia, you can't beat Holland and Frei."

I found myself thinking about the medical staff at our local family hospital—the ones who put Eric in a crib with the sides pulled up high and were so relieved when he headed to Buffalo for treatment.

"There was a real division back then, wasn't there?"

"What would irk me most about the local physicians or pediatricians," Sinks said, "was they were reluctant to deliver the hard news about the disease. Their education, their very practice didn't prepare them for how tough this effort was going to be. It wasn't unusual to have patients dumped on us at Roswell. Back in the '60s, pediatricians didn't like to deal with fatal diseases. It was a mind-set that they weren't prepared for and something frankly they didn't want to be involved in."

"Is that why you had so many foreign doctors rotate through? Two- and three-year postings?"

"In part, yes. At times I felt like I was running my own version of the United Nations. At one point, I even had two guys from Ireland, one Protestant and the other Catholic, and the fur would fly between those two. But I took a great deal of satisfaction out of working closely with my colleagues at Roswell Park because we shared a philosophy that we could make a difference, that some real results could be seen if we stayed after it. Back then we had people from around the world coming to Roswell Park to be a part of this. That was especially gratifying and difficult to pull off. I mean, we had doctors from overseas who were Muslim or

Jewish, Catholic, whatever kind of breakdown and background you wanted, we had it at Roswell. We were able to come together and help the kids. As long as we kept focused on the kids, progress was made."

The waiter arrived and I gingerly moved the texts to one side of the table, and there they sat, sort of a testament to what the leukemia doctors had been able to accomplish.

"But you must have had serious disagreements and arguments about treatment and procedures," I said.

"Certainly, we did," Sinks replied. "The ALGB, our main group, met several times a year and there was plenty of back and forth. But you had to give credit to Jim Holland for holding it all together. I began to call him Sam Rayburn. You remember Sam Rayburn, don't you?

"The congressman?

"The Speaker of the House for years and years. Jim had a lot of Sam Rayburn in him. He would sometimes hold a decisive vote on an important matter until late in the day when he knew he had the votes. Others may have left the meeting, heading home, only to find out we had moved ahead on some new treatment. Yes, Jim Holland knew how to get his way."

Throughout our lunch, I glanced several times at the books Sinks had brought me. They were impressive volumes, especially the one titled *Cancer Medicine* by Holland and Frei.

"So did Holland always carry the day?"

"Much of the time," Sinks said, "but there were some major disagreements."

"Was one of them about radiation?"

Sinks nodded and reached for the Holland and Frei book, flipping through to somewhere in the middle, pages he had already marked with a yellow sticky note.

"Like I said, I don't expect you to read all of this, but start here," he said and turned the book toward me. The chapter header read simply, "Acute Lymphoblastic Leukemia."

"Look this over and we'll talk about it next time."

17

Eric's outpatient progress record often read like postcards from a trip to a strange and distant land. In each one, his hemoglobin, white blood count, and platelets were recorded, in that order, on the next-to-last line, followed by the attending physician's signature. Even though his platelet count fluctuated from 47,500 to 567,500 (a platelet count of 150,000 to 400,000 is normal in children), a level of optimism crept into the official record. The acute lymphoblastic leukemia (ALL) was "in remission," read an entry for December 13, 1967. By the following entry, that diagnosis has been elevated to "complete remission."

"This healthy-looking boy returns for follow-up as scheduled . . . ," read the entry for January 3, 1968. "He was asymptomatic over the Christmas and New Year Holidays, except for a slight cough over the past three days, without fever or sputum."

A few weeks later: "This five-and-a-half-year-old boy returns to the clinic, healthy-looking without any complaints or symptoms."

By 1969, Eric's chemotherapy cocktail had shifted from maintenance doses of methotrexate to weekly IV doses of vincristine with prednisone, and daunomycin was back in play. Even though my brother was technically still in remission, the doctors at Roswell Park were determined to stay one step ahead of the cancer.

Everyone's fear was that it would find its way into the central nervous system in the spinal cord and brain.

"We knew the drugs were becoming more toxic and had to be carefully monitored," Mom said. "They weighed Eric every time he was at Roswell Park, sometimes twice a day, as they determined how much of these drugs they could use at a given time. They could only go so far in administering these drugs. And you would get results for a time. But you never knew how long. All of it was a dreaded mystery."

Eric continued to return to Roswell Park on a weekly, biweekly, or monthly basis, depending on the treatment and his condition. The scheduled outpatient visits, which sometimes required painful bone marrow tests, could stretch into several days if his blood cell and platelet numbers dipped too far. At the hospital and at home, the focus was on the here and now. We needed to be present, not put things off until tomorrow, because who knew what next week or next year might hold?

Back then I rarely asked questions about leukemia and Roswell Park. All I needed to know was that my brother was really sick. That was enough. Sometimes I would go in search of what I believed was normal, sometimes finding it at my friends' houses. I'd bike along the canal towpath to their homes and try to fall into those worlds. Their moms were almost always home, not making another trip to Buffalo for an outpatient visit. Dinner hit the table at 6 p.m. sharp—minutes after their dads came in the door from work. How I craved such convention and regularity at our house.

"You're going to live down in Olcott?" John asked.

"Just for the summer," I replied.

"But that's the best time of the year."

In our circle of friends, the ones who now rode the school bus a town over to Middleport, New York, and the junior-senior high school there, John Douglas was seen as something of a rebel and one who was ahead of his time. When the rest of us were still riding bikes on the canal towpath, John somehow pulled together enough secondhand parts to hot-wire a motorized scooter that he rode without a helmet. When we decided to start a garage band, which was envisioned as a blend of the Beatles and the Tijuana Brass, John's barn was where we rocked out until we agreed that the world wasn't ready for our attempt to reach the Top of the Pops.

John and I disagreed about the Vietnam War, which regularly led the nightly network news. Halfway around the world was nowhere to draw the line against communism, I told him. The country should cut its losses and get out while we could. But John wouldn't hear of it.

"Once you do that," he told me, "you never hear the end of it. Everybody will try to push you around."

And nobody pushed John Douglas around. Even though we were about the same height, on the runt end of the school pecking order, he never backed down from a confrontation and had gotten into his share of scraps at school. I usually looked for the door, avoiding such showdowns.

At Royalton-Hartland Central School, grades seven through twelve were under one roof, and some order was maintained by having the younger kids on the lower floors, where more teachers could keep an eye on us. Yet from the get-go, John ventured toward the top floor, almost looking for trouble among the juniors and seniors. He found it too. The buttonholes on the flannel shirts his mother bought him at Ames department store were often ripped because another upperclassman had grabbed him under the collar before John could push him away.

"When you leaving for the lake?" he asked.

"Right after school. We'll move back before school starts again."

We sat together on the bus that afternoon, pulling out of Middleport for the half-hour ride down Route 31 and home.

"Olcott's got to be a good 10 miles away." Too far for an unlicensed rider on a scooter made from junkyard parts.

"It's not far," I lied.

"Where you going to live?" he asked.

"In a house near the yacht club my dad joined. It's close to the boat too."

"Your dad must really love that boat," John said, looking out the window at the fields that would soon be filled with hay and corn. Even though it was only late April, the temperature was already climbing into the seventies. It promised to be a hot summer.

"And my mother is going to turn half of the house into a gift shop."

"A gift shop?"

"That's right. It'll be named Pick and Choose, and she's going to sell posters and cards, artwork that she saw last summer when we were up in Michigan."

John grew quiet, considering all of this. In a few minutes the bus would be at his house. My stop was another ten minutes farther west.

"Sometimes I cannot figure adults out," he said, almost to himself. "What makes them do the things they do?"

During that spring, Eric had been on a maintenance program of methotrexate and remained in remission. James Holland was in charge of the adult patients at the Buffalo campus and began to turn to daunomycin or daunorubicin. The drug could stymie cancer cells that could overwhelm the bone marrow. These so-called blast cells made it difficult to develop mature white blood cells. Holland had first heard about daunorubicin in the early 1960s when the French and the Italians worked with the drug.

Initially, Holland and Jerry Yates combined it and intravenous treatments of cytarabine or cytosine arabinoside (Ara-C), with promising results. After a second course of five days of Ara-C treatment and two days of daunorubicin, the patients often moved toward remission. But follow-up examinations of the bone marrow showed that 20 percent of the blast cells still remained. A similar problem was being seen on the children's side: patients could be put into remission, but how could they keep them there, especially knowing that if any cancer remained it would surely return?

With that in mind, Holland began a new clinical trial, with some fifty patients. With all of them, the blast cells lingered in the bone marrow after two rounds of the "five and two" treatments. That's when Holland and Yates decided to change things up. Instead of two rounds of "five and two," they went with a new regimen of seven days of Ara-C followed by three days of daunorubicin.

The first patient who participated in the "seven and three" treatment was a young woman with "a very aggressive acute leukemia," Holland recalled. She soon went into remission. More important, her bone marrow was clean. Subsequent studies tried ten days of Ara-C and three of daunorubicin. Other clinical trials added different chemotherapy drugs. None proved as effective as "seven and three," which soon became the industry standard.

Why did seven and three work better with patients than any other combination? To this day, nobody is completely sure, Yates said. "We treated patients with 'five and two' and it did not eliminate the leukemia in the majority of patients," he told me, "so we decided to try a few with 'seven and three' and found that for the majority of patients this seemed to do the trick."

But why?

Yates hesitated, not sure how to respond. "In the end, it doesn't matter, does it?" he answered. "The thing is that it worked, especially with older patients. That's what we were really focused on. We did what worked and kept moving ahead."

18

We soon realized that we had a good boat and a fine body of water on which to sail. Eight hundred feet at its deepest part, Lake Ontario held far more water than neighboring Lake Erie, the shallowest of the Great Lakes. Deeper waters meant that any sudden increase in wind was less likely to roil the waters—change a glassy surface into whitecap chop in a matter of minutes. Also, the shores of Lake Ontario are far less rocky than those of Superior, and the lake held fewer small islands and shallows than Lake Huron, so there was little reason to study elaborate charts and worry about running aground.

Moving ahead in this new world of ours became as comfortable as coming out of Olcott Harbor, rounding up into the prevailing westerly wind and letting that wide expanse of water, sometimes bottle green and other times a deeper shade of blue, stretch out ahead of us. To go all the way across Ontario, to reach the Canadian side and the city of Toronto, meant sailing in a northwesterly direction for about 40 miles. My father figured it would take seven to eight hours with a steady wind.

For some reason, I wasn't aboard that first trip across Lake Ontario. Instead I was at a state park outside of Coeur d'Alene, Idaho, attending the National Boy Scout Jamboree. There I crowded with other scouts around a small black-and-white television to watch Neil Armstrong and Buzz Aldrin walk on the moon. When I returned home, my siblings spoke in almost reverential tones about being so far out on the water and that moment when the American shore disappeared from view and there was nothing visible yet on the far horizon. One could steer by compass, following a specific heading, which was sometimes required because this was before the CN Tower and the skyscraper bank buildings were erected on the Canadian side, transforming that vista into something out of the Land of Oz.

"Dad just decided to go," Susan explained to me when I got home from Idaho.

"Maybe he was planning it for a while," Chris offered.

"But he never told any of us," Susan added.

"What was it like?" I asked, envious that I had missed out on such a family milestone.

"A lot of water," Susan said. "It can be a bit scary, being in the middle of the lake, with no land in sight."

"That Ontario is a big lake," Chris nodded. "But we made it back and Dad's already planning more trips. He and the little kids— Eric and Bryan—especially liked it."

"Everyone liked it," Susan said, "except maybe Mom."

So began the voyages from one shore to another, an arc between nations that required little paperwork or customs declarations decades before September 11, 2001. Really the only thing that was required was a good boat, a reasonably experienced crew, and the inclination to sail across so much open water in one fell swoop. If such matters had been put to a family vote, I wonder if the measure would have passed. But no family is a democracy, and Dad had decided we would be full-fledged sailors.

Accordingly, Dad devised a division of labor. As the oldest, I became the backup helmsman, and it was one of the best gifts he ever gave me. Dad taught me how to steer a boat, to be always conscious of the wind, realizing that such a force is never constant in direction or in magnitude—for steering a boat well has as much to do with feel as anything else. The breeze, fluctuating in direction and strength, is far from constant, never a given, and a good helmsman soon senses when a boat is going well. At such times in the thirteen-foot Nutshells, the smaller crafts we raced in junior sailing, you could actually hear the centerboard vibrate in its trunk below the waterline when the boat sped up. For the family trips, of course, we moved far beyond those dinghies in terms of weight and classification to yachts with lead keels weighing a ton or more. Still, the basic steering instincts remain the same. Watch the telltales to see when the wind shifts. Keep an eye on the leading edge of the jib, alert for a flutter or luff, especially when heading upwind. So much of sailing can be a mess of highfalutin jargon and technical terms. But when the wind begins to build, you learn to trust your gut and focus on the horizon.

Many of the yacht clubs that ring Lake Ontario have reciprocal visiting agreements in which members from one yacht club can stay overnight at another club for little cost. They are awarded slip space for the night and use of the facilities. Our Olcott Yacht Club was rarely a destination location. The shallow outdoor pool and aging bunkhouse paled in comparison to the luxurious clubs on the Toronto islands. For on the far side of Lake Ontario, there was Island Yacht Club, National, Queen City, and, the granddaddy of them all, the Royal Canadian Yacht Club (RCYC). The last one sported grass tennis courts and a bathhouse with monogrammed towels. On a trip to Toronto, we always headed first to RCYC. But so did every other visitor, especially on holiday weekends.

Slips and accommodations were on a first-come basis, and on one of those first crossings, by the time we reached Canada it was already dark and the RCYC harbormaster told us there was no room at the inn. In short order, we discovered that the rest of the Toronto Island yacht clubs were booked for the evening too.

"Do we need to go back home?" Chris asked.

Susan pointed out that there were plenty of other yacht clubs west of where we were, between Toronto and Hamilton, where the fires from the steel mills lit up the sky. But Dad ignored such suggestions. With little explanation, he told us to cast off and began to steer us across the busy harbor waters toward the Toronto skyline. We had no idea what he was up to as we drew closer to the busy city. Soon we heard the traffic noise echoing down to us from the elevated Queen Elizabeth Highway. Dad ordered us to tie all three of the white, pillow-like bumpers to the starboard side as he came up along the stone seawall near the flashing red-light sign for Tip Top Tailors.

"Are you sure we can be here?" Mom asked.

"If there's trouble, we'll just move along," he replied. "Any port in a storm, right?"

After we had secured the boat to the seawall, all of us grew quiet, listening to the cars racing by, the occasional siren, and the snippets of conversation that reached us across the stretch of darkening water.

"Don't worry," Dad said as Mom led the young ones down into the cabin for bedtime. "I'll stand guard, with the older kids."

Susan and I remained in the cockpit, and that evening I learned that a city, any large metropolis, can play with your mind. All the noise and confusion set the heart to racing at first. In time, though, once you begin to breathe easy again, many of the chaotic sounds become strangely reassuring. You settle into this particular moment and make your peace with it. Despite the novelty, you begin to sense that everything is going to be OK.

That's a fancy way of saying that I soon fell asleep that evening with the boat tied to the stone wall. Susan did, too, and we didn't awake until just before dawn when Dad needed help in casting off. As the others continued to sleep, we puttered back across Toronto harbor. The noise and commotion from the night before had almost disappeared. Instead, the whole world shimmered with first light, and the water was flat and smooth as far as we could see. Everything around us had been transformed into a vast mirror of water, on which our small boat caused only the faintest ripple.

Of all the voyages and crossings we made on Lake Ontario during our summers together, and they had to number in the hundreds before we all grew up and drifted into adulthood, that particular trip remains my favorite. On that evening, I first heard the echoes, even the call, of the big city. Our night docked in the shadow of the massive Tip Top Tailors sign demonstrated that we had become a pretty fair crew—even the regulars down at the yacht club would begrudgingly agree with that now. No matter what the wind brought our way, no matter how the situation played out, we could hang in the moment and somehow hold our own.

19

After moving to Memphis and building St. Jude Children's Research Hospital, Donald Pinkel began a methodical series of new clinical trials "based on all the stuff I knew, the experimental work and laboratory work and experience."

Pinkel called his approach Total Therapy and presented it to the ALGB group. He recalled that many of his peers said, "No, you can't do that." Yet Emil Frei "was not so much opposed, nor Jim Holland," Pinkel said. "But the others were not as brash and bold."

If you look at Pinkel's twenty-five years in Memphis, the treatments and procedures fall into four major stages or periods. The first ran from 1962 to 1966 and underscored that cancer-fighting drugs used in combinations worked far better than drugs used sequentially. Also, to overcome drug resistance, full-dosage chemotherapy was usually better than half-dosage amounts.

"Childhood lymphocytic leukemia can no longer be considered an incurable disease," Pinkel proclaimed in one paper. "Palliation is no longer a justifiable approach."

Indeed, in Memphis, Buffalo, and other hospitals across the country, more children with leukemia were moving into remission. The major obstacle had become how to keep them symptom-free. Too often the cancer returned, often with a vengeance. Studies by

Pinkel, Holland, and others revealed that leukemia patients, especially children, were developing meningeal leukemia in the central nervous system (CNS) soon after going into remission. With many patients, the chemotherapy drugs were too poorly diffused into the cerebrospinal fluid to be effective. As a result, the disease could linger in the CNS until it struck again.

"When you treat, you get rid of all systemic leukemia because it's drug-sensitive," Frei explained. "But our drugs didn't pass the blood–brain barrier. That is, they didn't get into the central nervous system."

The leukemia doctors tried to determine the best way to eradicate cancer cells in the CNS. Some advocated injecting more methotrexate and other chemotherapy drugs into the spinal canal, raising their levels in the cerebrospinal fluid. Early tests, though, showed that an appreciable amount still failed to pass through the blood–brain barrier.

At St. Jude, Pinkel began to administer varying degrees of radiation to the brain. Clinical trials in Memphis, given during what was called Era II (1967–1979), revealed that such treatments gave kids a better chance at long-term survival. Nearly 50 percent of the patients who had relapsed were soon called "long-term survivors." In fact, Pinkel was so encouraged after children had been in remission for several years that "we began stopping therapy, which was a very bold thing to do," he said. The doctors in Memphis ended maintenance measures to see if their patients would remain in remission. Amazingly, many did.

"It had never been done before," Pinkel later told Sue Banchich at Roswell Park. "So, by 1967, we were able to go out and say, 'It's not incurable. We can get one out of six children with ALL to go into remission, stay in remission, and stay in remission until we stop treatment. That was a big breakthrough.'"

Finding a cure had always been Pinkel's goal. "The development of effective therapy for children with acute lymphoblastic leukemia is one of the undisputed successes of modern clinical hematology," he wrote in 1993.

That said, Pinkel's aggressive approach sometimes made his colleagues in the ALGB uneasy. Decades later, James Holland told me that Pinkel "adopted the term Total Therapy from Sidney Farber with whom he had trained. It caused me, and perhaps others, some distress because the implication was that we were giving incomplete therapy. The use of cranial radiation was started by Pinkel while he was at Roswell. When he went to St. Jude, he continued it."

Radiation—how it should be used, if it should even be deployed at all against childhood leukemia—became a major topic of debate in the medical community. At St. Jude, radiation dosages of 500 to 1,200 rads "failed to reduce the frequency of CNS leukemia," an article authored by Pinkel and four others stated. So the amount of radiation was increased to 2,400 rads, but fewer than 9 percent of those patients achieved complete remission. In addition, 54 percent of the children who received 2,400 rads to the cranium and twice weekly treatments of methotrexate remained in "continuous complete remission for more than five years," the St. Jude group later wrote.

Despite such encouraging results, Pinkel's colleagues were concerned about the long-term impact of radiation on a patient's health. Holland's group in Buffalo published data indicating that children who received radiation to the brain lost IQ and that some showed "growth deficits" due to the effects on the pituitary gland.

"The cost of the cure," Sinks said. "That's something you hear a lot more about today. Many of us began to encounter it back in the '60s and '70s. What's best for the patient as you look toward the future? Back then, as now, it's not always an easy answer."

20

"How old were you when your brother died?" Pinkel once asked me.

"Seventeen."

We had been talking about how the doctor left Roswell Park to found St. Jude Children's Research Hospital in Memphis and how he decided to pursue Total Therapy.

"Seventeen," Pinkel repeated. "That's the kind of thing that can change a person's life. Tim, do you have any children yourself?"

"A daughter and a son. They're both grown now."

"And your brother's death? How did that influence you as a parent?" Somehow Pinkel's interest, his bedside manner, had turned the tables on this conversation. Now he was interviewing me.

"Deep down it scared me," I admitted. "I never felt more vulnerable until I became a father."

"That's understandable."

"It probably didn't help that my son, my youngest, looked a lot like my brother when he was a baby. He outgrew a lot of those characteristics, but for a time it would stop some family members in their tracks."

After we hung up, our conversation kept rumbling around inside my head. How much had my brother's death affected me as a person, as a parent? I had never talked that much about my brother to my own kids. In large part that was because I had known so little about the medicines he was on and the procedures he was subjected to until I began this search to find the doctors who had treated him and other children like him.

To be honest, though, I hardly mentioned Eric to my own daughter and son because, deep down, I was afraid. Afraid of what would happen if they ever came down with such a cruel illness. For I'd seen how much such a disease can weigh on parents. How much easier it was to be a big brother rather than a father in such situations. As a sibling, I could shut everything out, or at least try to. How much better to try and keep the past at arm's length and move ahead, as fast as we can, across another stretch of open water.

On Lake Ontario, we began to excel as a family, calling out the next wind shift, ready to drop one sail and run up another stretch of fabric. That said, you cannot outrun every squall line, steer clear of every storm that comes your way.

One time, coming back from Canada, the seas became rough in a hurry when we were still far from shore. Even though it was pretty warm, Eric huddled with Mom under a blanket while she gave him crackers and ginger ale. She was determined that he keep something down.

"It was not unusual to hit rough weather, or to get seasick, but we were usually counseled to stare at the horizon to get our bearings or told to go down below and close our eyes," my sister Susan said. "If you were really struggling, Dad would have you take the helm and the combination of watching the horizon and having an actual responsibility would either cure you or give you something else to think about.

"That day Mom was desperate to keep something in Eric because he was approaching dehydration. This was not ordinary seasickness.

It was a reaction to a change in his medication. On another crossing, we might have changed course for a smoother ride, or turned back and tried another day. But with Eric in the condition he was in, the only thing left to do was to keep him hydrated and reach shore, get home to Olcott, as soon as we could.

"So that's what we did. Mom nursed and Dad sailed."

Together we rode out another storm, and several hours later, wet and bedraggled, we dropped the sails and, with the engine now on, made the sweeping turn between the bookend brown-metal piers that mark the entrance to Olcott Harbor. Somehow we had made it home.

21

Decades later, my own son, Chris, was often sick as a young boy. His ailments were never as serious as leukemia, but he suffered from viral-induced asthma for years. That's how I found myself back in the land of hospitals and doctors, and, I'll be honest, it soon unnerved me.

"Are you all right?" Jacqui asked on our first trip to the emergency room at the University of Michigan medical complex.

It was late autumn in 1995, and we had moved to Michigan for the school year, with me on a Knight-Wallace journalism fellowship. Back home in the Washington, D.C., area, where Chris had been born, he had been a colicky baby at first. Still, he soon outgrew the hours of crying to become a happy-go-lucky kid. He loved sports, being outside, trying to keep up with the bigger kids. That's where he could often be found until a dry, raspy cough, which began deep down in his lungs, forced him to come inside. That cough was the kind of sound that a parent soon learned to dread.

"This place gives me the willies," I told my wife and glanced around us. The gleaming hallways seemed to lead off in all directions from the waiting room, like we were on the edge of an elaborate maze.

"Why's that?"

"It reminds me too much of my brother."

That evening Chris was given Albuterol to relax the muscles in his lungs and increase the airflow when he breathed. Eventually he would be on a wide range of medicines, including Singulair and Asmanex. We bought a nebulizer, a compact machine with a face mask that made a hissing sound as it turned the Albuterol into a fine mist that could be absorbed deeper into the lungs. All along, the doctors tried to reassure us. After all, Chris was barely three years old. In all likelihood, he would outgrow this condition. While I nodded appreciatively at such advice, late at night, when everyone else was asleep, I would sometimes tiptoe into my son's bedroom and rest my hand lightly on his back. What concerned me was how still I had to stand, barely breathing myself, to feel any appreciable rise and fall in his small body.

That fall in Ann Arbor, on Halloween, Chris was so sick with the asthma that he couldn't go out with the other kids for regular tricks and treats. We were living that year in married student housing at the University of Michigan. The cough had returned with the onset of the colder weather. Despite being sick, Chris didn't want to miss out on Halloween, and I couldn't blame him. After all, I also had fond memories of high jinks on that evening.

Late that afternoon, we took him to the university clinic nearby, and the nurse who examined him said he could go out as long as he didn't overexert himself. Back home, with night coming on, we discussed what costume could work for a kid who had to stay in a stroller. After bundling Chris up in several layers of clothes to keep him warm, we went with a blue Michigan windbreaker, with a pillow stuffed underneath. A ball cap with that distinctive block M and a whistle and cord completed the look. For Chris was now Bo Schembechler, legendary Wolverine football coach, with me pushing him around the neighborhood. The costume was a hit, and

Chris raked in as much candy as any kid on North Campus that evening.

Just before Christmas, Chris had another bad bout of asthma. (We would later discover that fresh-cut evergreen trees set him off.) We had driven a few hours east, across the Canadian border, to spend the holiday with my wife's mother. Her house was decked out for the season, looking like something from a Norman Rockwell painting.

That evening, however, Chris's cough returned. I'm the light sleeper in our household, and I stole down to the small room where my son was at rest. The dry rasp grew in frequency and ferocity, a monster, something evil that boiled up from deep inside of him. I sat beside his bed, stroking his head, wishing I could somehow lift the illness free from his small body. Take it and make it mine.

Soon I awoke Jacqui, and we bundled Chris up for another trip to the emergency room. Dressed in his snow jacket, zipped up to the chin, with hat and mitts on, Chris gazed out the back window at the holiday lights as we sped along Lakeshore Boulevard in the predawn darkness. I glanced at him in the rearview mirror, praying that he would be all right.

At the hospital, another face mask was placed over his nose and mouth, and he was told to try and relax, to breathe deeply. As he tried to do so, a young doctor, a woman maybe in her early thirties, placed the stethoscope to his chest and back, and listened intently.

It was Christmas Eve morning, and few pharmacies were open. So as soon as Chris stabilized, I headed to the CVS farther up Lakeshore Boulevard, closer toward Toronto, to fill the prescriptions. Driving along, I was tired and worried, and with my mind elsewhere, I ran a red light, turning the wheel violently to the left to barely avoid an onrushing car. The near miss was so sudden that our Subaru wagon conked out, coming to a rest in the middle of the intersection before I could crank over the engine and again be on my way.

When I returned to the hospital, the assortment of meds secure in my coat pocket, I saw Jacqui talking with the young doctor outside the examination room. "She says we should be giving Chris more of the medicine," Jacqui said, "especially the Albuterol."

"But other doctors—" I began.

"I cannot speak to that," the doctor said.

She looked like she had been up for hours. With dark circles under tired eyes, she undoubtedly wanted to finish her shift and go home for the holiday. Yet she had stayed to speak with us—to urge us to try a different approach with our son.

"The meds he's being given are good ones," she said in a weary voice. "I just think they are being started too late with him. By the time he's on the Albuterol, for example, the asthma has settled into the lungs. Can I make a suggestion?"

We both nodded.

"As soon as he begins to cough, start him on the Albuterol. He can be on Singulair and other drugs for maintenance too, but starting the Albuterol right away should help with the more serious symptoms."

Jacqui and I looked at each other. The other doctors that Chris had seen, the ones on the other side of the border, had never been this explicit or aggressive.

"You have a nebulizer?" she asked.

"We just bought one," answered Jacqui.

"Use it," the young doctor said. "Bring it with you on family vacations from now on. It becomes another piece of luggage for you. I'll write you a script for more Albuterol vials, so you'll have plenty of them."

"He hates that face mask," I said.

"Sing to him, stroke his head," the doctor said. "Get as much of that medicine into his lungs as you can when he starts to cough."

By that afternoon, we had taken Chris back to the holiday house in Oakville, just past Bronte Harbor, one of the ports I used to sail to as a kid, and there the countdown to Christmas was well under way. Jacqui and I talked about what the doctor had advised. Although we eventually forgot the doctor's name, we would follow her recommendations for years to come.

22

"I wish he wouldn't play," Dad said.

"Does it really make a difference?" Mom replied. "With what he's going through up at Roswell, he's tough enough."

"But still . . ."

The two of them were in the kitchen, talking softly. The new hockey season, another round of tryouts, was only a few days away. I sat on the stairs, eavesdropping on their conversation.

My father had led us down the waters of Lake Ontario, our inland sea, but I was the one who took us to the rink, the sheet of ice for our winters together. I remember the exact moment when I fell in love with the game of hockey. Dad and I were returning from Lockport on a Saturday afternoon in early May, driving east out of town on East Avenue, which became Route 31, heading toward Rochester. It was spring 1967, and Eric was home from Roswell Park. Dad had the radio set to the CBC out of Toronto.

Our home on Canal Road was almost in the shadow of the Niagara Escarpment, that ridge of land that runs west to east across Niagara County and forms the world-famous Falls. Coming out of town, Route 31 follows the escarpment, which allowed us to hear the Toronto radio stations on the far side of Lake Ontario.

The Niagara Escarpment actually begins in Wisconsin, on the far west side of Lake Michigan, and runs in a half-circle, almost like an upside-down smile, as it sweeps into Canada. Near Hamilton, Ontario, it straightens out into a horizontal map line of dolomite limestone, extending across our part of the world until it tapers away to nothing near Watertown, New York, north of Syracuse.

The formidable ridge of land doesn't exist along any fault line, and near as geologists can tell, the escarpment was formed by unequal erosion, in which different rocks weathered away and others proved to be more resistant over millions of years. Such a hypothesis doesn't seem to justify something so significant, however. For instance, Niagara Falls doesn't exist without the escarpment to plunge over. Without this ridge of land, Father Louis Hennepin, perhaps the first white man to see the roaring cataract, doesn't fall to his knees in prayer when he bears witness to one of the natural wonders of the world. In our household, the Niagara Escarpment came into play almost every day. We drove up and down its flanks going in and out of town. The land divide influenced what we watched on TV and listened to on the radio. In the days before cable television and the Internet, we soon learned that to the north were the Toronto stations: CBC with *Hockey Night in Canada* and CHUM-FM with its rock music. To the southwest were WGR and WKBW, the Buffalo stations, and at night, if one fiddled with the dial on the transistor radio, WJR, "The Great Voice of the Great Lakes," out of Detroit. Rarely could we pick up all those signals at once. Reception depended on the weather, time of the year, and how close we were to the Niagara Escarpment.

On this Tuesday evening, the CBC was airing playoff hockey, the Stanley Cup Finals between the Montreal Canadiens and the hometown Maple Leafs. Despite being the underdogs, the Leafs were ahead three games to two and ahead by a goal, with time running down in game six.

For some reason, Dad pulled over to the side of the road after we turned onto Day Road, which led down to our house. There we sat for a few minutes as the announcer, Foster Hewitt, called the action late in the third period. In my mind, I could picture the teams moving back and forth, the capacity crowd at the old Gardens in Toronto on its feet, as the remaining seconds counted down to this improbable triumph. The Canadiens' roster had Jean Beliveau, Yvan Cournoyer, and Henri Richard—the pride of French-speaking Canada. If the Leafs could hang on, they would be the oldest team to win the Cup, with an average player age of thirty-one years old.

In the closing seconds, the Canadiens made rush after rush toward the Toronto net, using their superior speed. The Leafs did their best to blunt such attacks while goalie Terry Sawchuk, who had begun the series as the backup, battled to keep the puck out of the net.

Together Dad and I sat in the front seat of the family station wagon, listening to the game end, smiling at each other as the cheers at Maple Leaf Gardens grew louder. Then it was over. Toronto scored an empty net goal and captured the championship. Dad put the car in gear and headed down the steep hill, leading to the Erie Canal and the remaining mile or so to home.

When the next season began in October, I was regularly watching *Hockey Night in Canada* on Saturday evenings, and when a new rink, the Kenan Arena, opened in town, I decided to try out even though I could barely skate at the time. After I made it through my first year playing organized hockey, my brother Chris followed me into the game, becoming a solid defenseman. Soon Eric and Bryan were old enough to play in the Mite Division, the youngest age group.

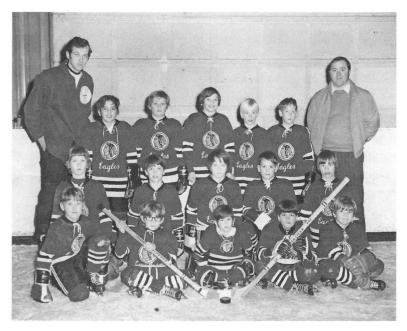

Eric, middle of the second row, on the Lockport Mite hockey team.

"I worry about Eric getting hurt," Dad said. "I mean hockey? That can be as rough as football."

"And none of them will ever play football," Mom told him. "That's where we draw the line."

"But we'll let them play hockey?"

"We did with the first two. We can't exactly say it's OK for Tim and Chris and then tell the other two no."

"But Eric's the one I worry about."

"I know, but he's doing fine. The sessions at Roswell Park are going well. He wants to be like his brothers, do what they're doing. Sometimes that's what keeps him going through all of this."

Reluctantly Dad agreed that Eric and Bryan would play on the same Mites team that first year. Eric was six and Bryan was five years old, and they were put on a line with a kid named Barney, who eventually became a topflight goalie. Mom explained to the coaches that Eric was "a bleeder." That he had leukemia and would likely miss parts of the season due to his ongoing treatments at Roswell Park. Eric maneuvered about the ice with an almost robotic cadence. (Bryan was faster and better able to join the fray.) Eric wore no. 3, and Mom later told me it was because he had three brothers.

"Brothers who gave him strength, egged him on, and had so much fun dreaming of possibilities," she said.

Eric and I played the same position—left wing. For anyone new to the game, wobbly on his skates and unsure of where he was supposed to be, wing is an ideal place to be on the ice. The position requires little defensive responsibility, and one can look to score. That said, neither Eric nor I scored many goals back then.

At the time, Eric was on a maintenance schedule of methotrexate (30 milligrams biweekly), with "pulsating doses" of vincristine, which was alternated with daunomycin and augmented by prednisone. This particular chemotherapy cocktail had kept him technically in remission for almost two years. The methotrexate was given via injections into the spine, while the daunomycin was applied by intravenous injection. Despite the regular trips to Roswell Park, Eric played on and soon became a part of one of the great moments in family hockey lore.

It was a Saturday afternoon in February and the Mites had to be playing Depew. It seemed that the Lockport teams were always playing the Depew Saints in those days because the rival rinks were less than 20 miles away from each other, a straight shot up Transit Road.

The Saints had come to the Kenan Center on this day and sported an impressive first line, centered by a big kid who could really skate. Eric and Bryan didn't see much action back then. Still, when they got on the ice, they tried their best, and by this point in the season, their line had even gained a nickname—the Mighty Mites.

Coach Doug Puff played them only a few times a period and looked to match them up against the opposition's weaker skaters. Among most teams, especially at this age, there was an unspoken agreement: the best players played against the best and the weakest against the rest. Despite this gentleman's pact, midway through the second period against Depew, the Mighty Mites were caught on the ice for several minutes, with no whistles for offsides or icing to facilitate a substitution. Sensing an advantage, the Saints' coach changed his forwards on the fly, not waiting for another stoppage in play. As Eric and Bryan struggled to return to their bench, Depew's top line, with the big kid at center, gained possession of the puck and turned up ice, streaking toward the Lockport end of the ice.

As the Mighty Mites retreated to the sidelines, they found themselves on a collision course with the Saints' top line. Eric made contact first, bouncing off one of the Depew forwards and falling down in a heap. Bryan and Barney trailed him, and they somehow sandwiched the hotshot center. Even though they barely came up to the kid's chest, they slowed him down enough so that the Depew star lost the puck.

Dad, Chris, and I were watching together, right up against the Plexiglas near the spectator bleachers.

"Look out now," Dad said, and behind us we heard the parents, perhaps thirty or more, rise as one and shout in unison. All eyes were on the three Mites as they battled Depew's star player.

The big kid shoved Bryan, who rolled off from him like snow falling from a steep-pitched roof. In response, Barney pushed back, but to no avail. Behind the fracas, Eric was on all fours, try-ing to retrieve his stick. He appeared to be out of the play until Bryan went at the star center one last time, causing the kid to slide backward, where he smacked into Eric.

In a scene right out of the Marx Brothers or the Three Stooges, the Depew star lost his balance and toppled over Eric, landing flat on his back. Seeing their chance, Bryan and Barney fell on top of him, pinning the Saints' best player down in front of his bench.

The referee blew his whistle and helped everyone untangle. In another game, he could have easily called a penalty or two. But trying to swallow a smile, he ushered the players back to their re-spective benches as many in the crowd cheered the Mighty Mites' effort.

"That's what I call teamwork," Dad said.

As MUCH AS we chased the promise of open water and a wide hori-zon, we had a fair-sized country pond a short walk from our back-yard.

When I was Eric's age, Grandpa Lee operated a sand and gravel pit on a piece of land he owned beyond the railroad tracks in back of our house. At its height, a three-bay garage and several dump trucks and a bulldozer were housed there, with workmen on-site throughout the summer months. The first time I ever rode shot-gun on a dozer was back at the gravel pit. I was six years old, al-ready being groomed as the successor in the engineering company that my grandfather had founded before World War II, the firm my father had helped grow when he was called home from the University of Michigan.

The small quarry did a brisk business until they hit water one summer afternoon. Soon the earthen bowl, 30 feet tall in places, began to fill. The water was on them so quickly that a dump truck or two was supposedly abandoned there, left to rust in an underwater grave.

Over the years, the new lake continued to grow gradually. There used to be a small island, where Grandpa Lee took Chris and me in a wooden rowboat. We paddled about, fishing for perch and blue gill, which had been stocked in the new pond, before taking a break on the island in the center of it all. There we would start a fire, Huck Finn style, and roast hot dogs in the shadow of the escarpment and Route 31.

After relocating to Lake Ontario to sail, we didn't spend many more summer afternoons at Wendel Pond, as the locals began to call it. Yet in the winter, the pint-sized lake became our favorite place for pond hockey.

We had first tried the Erie Canal, across the road from our house, but the current, even in the dead of winter, made for rough patches of ice. Just past the bridge that the Penguin's mast couldn't fit underneath was a smaller pond on Groff Road. Cattails lined the shoreline, similar to the ponds where Lucius Sinks had learned to skate as a kid. But if we had a big game, the place to play was Wendel Pond. If the snow wasn't too deep, we would pack everybody into my mother's station wagon, and I'd drive past the concrete-block garage where the evacuation machinery had once been housed. Over the years, vandals had broken several of the plate-glass garage windows, and in the warmer months, the shards scattered across the ground glittered like pirates' silver.

Once we reached the pond, we shoveled off a stretch of clear ice, and the kids in the houses up along Route 31 would come down, too. Our patch of ice, the outdoor rink itself, depended on how many of us showed up. One Sunday afternoon in January, when the sun came out, we had thirty kids of all ages there. The setup was so large that we had one area for the game, with the snow pushed up high along the sides, and another, smaller area where newcomers warmed up, practicing their skating and stick-handling, before coming in.

There was no lifting the puck because we never had bona fide goalies for such games. No checking, either. Instead, everyone played about everywhere, a swirl of players, and it was a game that emphasized passing and skating. Depending on the wind direction, we would switch ends and change up teams whenever the game became too lopsided. We tested the ice by throwing a large stone or one of the cement blocks from the old garages onto the ice. If it could take that weight, it could take ours. We talked about forming a human ladder if there ever was a massive crack and somebody fell in. But, thankfully, we never had to deploy those emergency tactics.

I wasn't a very good player on indoor ice back then. During one early morning practice at the Kenan Center, the coach kept running the same breakout play over and over again, and I never did get it right. Yet outdoors, on the pond, nobody cared about position responsibility or any overall game plan. The biggest disaster came when the puck was lost in a snowdrift, so we learned to bring along a few. On the pond, we could play for hours, trying a new skill like skating backward, shifting the puck from forehand to backhand. Only when it got too cold or too dark or we finally ran out of pucks did we head for home.

By Eric's second season of organized hockey, he had lost much of his hair due to another round of chemotherapy. He didn't think much of it until he walked into the locker room at the Kenan Arena one Saturday morning and his teammate Frankie exclaimed, "Your hair's gone."

Eric told him it was because of "some dumb medicine. It'll grow back." But Frankie and others on the team continued to stare at him.

Later that afternoon, when Mom came to pick him up, he told her, "My bald head scares people. Maybe I should get a wig."

The two of them picked one out and trimmed it to fit his head. The wig lasted until the first hot days of summer when we went swimming at our Aunt Marguerite's. She had a small pool in her backyard, and Eric jumped right in. As he sank underwater, the wig plopped to the surface, floating there until Eric retrieved it. The rest of us began to giggle as he put it back on his head. But when it floated free again, he began to laugh too. Soon he tossed the wig on to the pool deck. There it sat for the rest of the day, and even though it came home with us, my brother rarely bothered with the wig again.

23

By spring 1970, James Holland's group had gained national attention. What began as a handful of hospitals in the effort against cancer had grown to twenty-six facilities with 167 physicians as members and five foreign countries represented. The ALGB was making progress, so much so that *Look* magazine assigned Roland H. Berg to do a major feature on the effort and specifically Roswell Park. The headline would be: "We Have a Chance to Beat Leukemia Now."

Berg had written a book about polio and the Salk vaccine, and a decade earlier as a press officer with the National Foundation for Infantile Paralysis, he had nearly become the first one to write at length about Henrietta Lacks and how her cells launched a multi-million-dollar industry.

"That *Look* article was a big deal for Roswell Park," Lucius Sinks said. "The doctors probably didn't care that much. We were focused more on the day to day, but for the others at the hospital, they were happy to get the recognition."

Berg spent nearly a week at Roswell Park conducting interviews, and the story ran over five pages, with seven black-and-white photographs, on May 5, 1970. Joan Baez, the folk singer, and her husband, David Harris, were on the cover of the issue, and the story

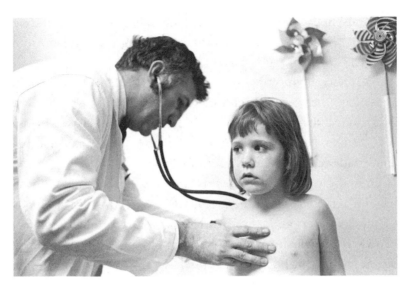

Dr. Lucius Sinks with a young patient. John Vachon, *Look* magazine, 1970.

inside detailed the couple's last days together before Harris left for jail in his protest of the Vietnam War. Other cover headlines included "A Year with the Queen," an excerpt from a new book about Great Britain's Queen Elizabeth, and "Nixon's Big Gamble," an inside report about the president's political strategy with minority groups. Yet no words in this issue of *Look* were as audacious as the subhead for Berg's story about Roswell Park and the doctors there. "A fatal disease shows signs of yielding to a cooperative plan of treatment. As more children survive, scientists predict that cure is now a realistic target," it reads.

Even in the midst of such optimism and newfound notoriety, Jimmie Holland, James Holland's wife and a noted doctor herself, wondered whether the members of ALGB were overlooking the patients' mental states in the campaign against cancer. Such concerns arose during after-work gatherings in the kitchen of the

Hollands' house in north Buffalo. If any members of ALGB were in town, they were invited to stop by, joining the regulars from Roswell Park.

"We ended up meeting so much in our kitchen because back in those days there weren't a lot of restaurants in Buffalo. Plus, we had young kids," Jimmie Holland said. "So it just made more sense for Jim to invite everyone over from Group B, and I'd make something and everyone could relax and talk."

Jimmie Holland remembered Emil Frei and Donald Pinkel around her kitchen table discussing various treatments with many of the doctors from Roswell Park. One such evening, she asked, "You guys do a battery of tests for the physical ailments, but do you ever find out how the patients feel about what you're doing to them?"

The doctors answered no. They were too busy saving lives. Feelings, emotions, the mental state of affairs? They would catch up to such aspects of care once they had put more patients into remission.

"Their reaction was something like, 'Well, they'll feel better once we find a cure,'" Jimmie Holland recalled. "I couldn't help thinking that there was more to focus on there."

Jimmie Holland had grown up in Nevada, Texas, about 50 miles northeast of Dallas, during the Great Depression. She enjoyed taking care of sick animals as a kid and graduated from high school as World War II ended. At first, Jimmie Holland was going to be a nurse, but she soon realized that she could do more as a doctor. She went to Baylor University in Waco and afterward Baylor's medical school in Houston, where she was one of three women in a class of nearly ninety.

"Three women, three Jews—the usual quota for Texas," she recalled.

That said, Jimmie Holland remembered that it "was a great time to be in school because everybody wanted to learn, to make up for lost time," she said. "The GIs were returning from the war, so you got caught up in that too."

Her original plan was to return to Texas after a rotation in psychiatry in St. Louis, followed by a residency in Boston in 1955 during the polio epidemic. Yet Holland never came home to practice. On a visit to Buffalo to see a friend who was a surgical fellow at Roswell Park, she met James Holland, and they soon married.

After one evening playing hostess for the gatherings that had become nicknamed "the kitchen think tank," Jimmie Holland asked her husband if he would help her start a committee to study how and what cancer patients felt during treatments—the mental side of things. In those days, she was working part-time at the University of Buffalo's School of Medicine and as the head of psychiatry at Erie County Medical Center. That said, everyone knew that the real advances against cancer were being made at Roswell Park. James Holland gave his blessing, and Jimmie Holland became one of the founders of psychological oncology, or psycho-oncology, a subspecialty that explores the psychological, social, behavioral, and ethical aspects of cancer.

One of her early patients summed up the need for such an approach. "They have measured everything but my thoughts and mind," Holland quoted him in her book, *The Human Side of Cancer*. "Somehow, my mental attitude, the stress, the anguish should be analyzed and studied the same as my physical condition."

In the years after the conversations around her kitchen table in Buffalo, Jimmie Holland wrote the first textbook on psycho-oncology and started the psychiatry service at Memorial Sloan-Kettering Cancer Center in New York in 1977. In addition, in 1994 she received the highest award of the American Cancer Society, the Medal of Honor.

"Of course, the wheels aren't put in motion without Jim's help," Holland said. "My husband was able to approve the idea and away I went. In looking back on it, I found my heart in Buffalo, at least in a professional sense. That's where I was able to explore how people can manage catastrophic illness. I found that I could help them do so."

Jimmie Holland added that the campaign against cancer, especially childhood leukemia, changed when patients "began to survive this disease. That goes back to the great work that Jim and the others were doing. And it sure made it easier to talk about cancer. Betty Ford and Happy Rockefeller were very public about their breast cancer. We had a popular movie in *Love Story*, which was about leukemia. It was a good time to join the effort in my own way."

In doing so, Holland and others broadened the effort against cancer, putting the focus on patient care as much as finding a cure. She defines "palliative care" as any procedure that provides "comfort and [is] not focused on cure of the disease."

According to the National Cancer Institute, palliative care is now "given throughout a patient's experience with cancer. It should begin at diagnosis and continue through treatment, follow-up care, and the end of life." Such measures are given in addition to cancer treatment today, and "when a patient reaches a point in which treatment to destroy the cancer is no longer warranted, palliative care becomes the total focus of care."

This policy represents a major shift from the mid-1960s, as finding the balance between medical treatments and a patient's quality of life continues today. "When it comes to cancer care in this country, we know how to help each other to keep fighting," a health care expert told me, "but how do we know when to stop? When is enough enough?"

I can count on both hands the number of times that we, as a family, visited 5 East Unit, where the children with leukemia were housed at Roswell Park. My brother, as Mom reminded us, lived in two worlds. When things were going well, he was home at Canal Road and at Olcott with us. When his health suffered, he needed to spend more time in Buffalo, at the hospital that made me uneasy, with its long hallways and hushed conversations.

Dr. Martin Brecher recalled that there was "only one private room" on the twelve-bed unit when my brother was a patient at Roswell Park. So, when a parent stayed "overnight with a child (something that was not encouraged then, although it is today), they would be sleeping in a room with other patients and, possibly, other patients' family members. This was certainly not conducive to privacy."

My parents were the only ones in our family ever to stay overnight with Eric. The rest of us would visit for much of a day if he was unable to be home with us. Once Susan, Chris, and I happened on the Cigarette Hall of Fame, which was located on a lower floor. Here, framed photographs of celebrities lined the walls—famous names who had died of lung cancer and other diseases attributable to smoking. We recognized Nat "King" Cole, one of Mom's favorite singers. A small legend stated he had died of lung cancer at the age of forty-five. Nearby hung portraits of Humphrey Bogart (fifty-seven, throat cancer), Walt Disney (sixty-five, lung cancer), Buster Keaton (seventy, emphysema), and more.

"But Eric's never smoked," Chris said.

"He has a different kind of cancer," Susan said.

"Grandpa Lee's told me never to smoke," I added. "He says it's the one thing he couldn't kick, even if he had all the tea in China."

"He told me the same thing," Susan said, eyeing the rows of photographs. "And he's right about that."

"Then why do they have all these pictures in this hospital?" Chris asked.

"Because studies have shown that people who smoke are more likely to get cancer," Susan added. "Lung cancer, throat cancer, emphysema, heart disease—all the ones that are listed here. They established the link between smoking and those diseases."

Chris nodded. "So Eric's different?"

"That's right," Susan told us. "They haven't pinned down the cause yet. They haven't gotten it really figured out, like they have with smoking."

The three of us stood together and gazed down the corridor lined with photographs of the rich and famous.

"I hope they figure it out soon," Chris said.

By this time, Dad had cobbled together enough money to buy a modest three-bedroom house with an overgrown yard and bandstand-like gazebo in Olcott (population 2,000 during the summer months). It was a few blocks from the yacht club and the stone-pebble beach near the harbor piers. To the delight of us kids, it was around the corner from George's Market, which offered a fantasy land of such delicacies as Bazooka Joe bubble gum, Slim Jim sticks, and Mrs. Smith's fruit pies. For kids who had grown up in the country, miles away from the nearest town, Olcott was a bustling metropolis. The oldest of us brought our bikes from home and ventured forth from our new beachhead on the south shore of Lake Ontario.

To this day, I'm not sure why one day I decided to bike up West Main Street, past Jackson Street, turning right on Crescent Heights toward the West Bluff. The narrow street runs along Lake Ontario, flanked by summer cottages and a few year-round establishments. Down at the harbor, Susan, Chris, and I participated in junior sailing at the yacht club, and we were regularly on the water by 9 a.m., racing beyond the metal piers that marked the entrance to Olcott harbor. We would swim in the small yacht club pool, where I would later lifeguard, or even jump into Lake Ontario itself from the left-side pier, with the small tower and the red blinking light, the same one we searched for when heading home after another family voyage.

I had heard there were other kids about, ones my age that didn't sail with the junior sailors or belong to the yacht club. They were out there, perhaps on the West Bluff. So one afternoon, after the 13-foot Nutshell sloops we used for junior sailing were stored away, I biked up West Main. With the breeze coming off the lake, it was considerably cooler than down on Van Buren Street. Many places had fair-sized lawns, and some featured paved driveways with basketball hoops hanging from the garage roofs. I pedaled along the West Bluff, envious of such things, when I heard kids yelling and cheering not too far up the road. As I drew closer, I realized it was infield chatter, something heard only on a ball diamond.

Rolling out to my left, in a sunken field by an orchard of dwarf apple trees, kids were playing softball. The field featured plenty of quirks and idiosyncrasies. Home plate had been set up in the far corner, near the first row of fruit trees, with the infield of weathered bases. Just beyond that regular configuration, left field arose on an incline all the way to the street, where I watched astride my yellow Schwinn bike. Center field was regulation enough, before it began to fall away to the right, leading downhill until a half-foot drop-off marked the far property line.

As I watched, one of the older boys, a kid with muscular arms and hair almost as dark as mine, turned nicely on a pitch, pulling it up the left-field hill, toward me. The infielders watched it soar over their heads and the shortstop, the tallest on the opposing team, ran only a few steps up the hill before letting the ball hit and roll back to him. By deploying such local knowledge, he held the batter to a long single.

After three outs, as they changed sides, somebody noticed me up on the street.

"You want to play?"

"I don't have my glove," I replied.

"You can borrow one. C'mon."

I walked my bike down the hill and laid it in the grass beside the others near the third-base line.

"I'm Burg," said the kid with dark hair, who was about my size. "That's Danny Clogston and his little brother. And those are the Stein boys out in the field. Go with them. They're getting killed today."

Somebody tossed me a glove, and I pulled it over my left hand, trying to smooth out the pocket so it felt more comfortable. Soon enough everything fell into the rhythm of another game. The next day, I convinced my brother Chris to tag along with me. Within the week, we were regulars, playing ball on the West Bluff. After dinner, the adults set up lawn chairs on the side of the street and watched our titanic struggles until darkness fell. Sometimes Dad stopped by after work on the pretense of making sure we got home all right.

For a time, summer fell into an idyllic routine. Weekday mornings we sailed with the club juniors, and late in the afternoons we played ball up on West Bluff. On the weekends, we often went for another cruise on Lake Ontario, regularly crossing over to the Canadian side.

Being out on the water almost every day, we learned to look to the treetops to read the wind—determining its strength and direction. Even if the lake spread out like a huge mirror, flat as a pancake toward Ontario's far shore, with only the faintest ripple of waves rolling up the flat stone beach near Olcott's twin piers, we knew that, if there was a rustle in the leaves high up, more wind was on the way. Things were about to change again.

On the water, we soon learned that conditions were never the same. Sometimes the wind would be ripping as soon as we cleared Olcott's piers, with white caps breaking like distant explosions well offshore. Other times, the breeze would die down to nothing as we moved away from the American shore, leaving us almost motionless, stranded in a stretch of flat water for as far as the eye could see.

As much as Dad listened to the local weather reports, going so far as to buy a shortwave radio, the lake itself remained the wild card, the joker in the deck for every family trip. No matter how much information one gathered beforehand, it didn't matter until we were out on the water, seeing everything firsthand.

The most promising crossing to the other side could unravel due to the lack of wind, leaving us in the middle of this wide expanse of blue-green, going so slow that a cracker or part of a sandwich thrown into the water when our father wasn't looking would bob along, neck and neck with us. That's what made the days when it blew hard even more stunning. The swells built, one upon the other, and we were forced to pull down sails, feeling the boat pitch and fall as the next series of waves assaulted us. Were we ever scared? Sure. By then, we were a family of six kids and two adults on a sailboat that was never longer than thirty feet, going across a Great Lake with an average depth of 283 feet, second only to Lake Superior.

One weekend, my brother Chris and I joined Dad's crew for a race from Youngstown to Bronte Harbor, almost due north across Lake Ontario on the Canadian shore. The day had brought rain, fog, and fickle winds upon us. We didn't do well, finishing far back in the pack. We crossed the finish line in the dark, dropped the sails, and motored for the small cove where the racers were scheduled to spend the night.

As we approached Bronte Harbor, wisps of fog drifted toward us, soon engulfing us. As we passed the blinking red light to this harbor in silence, none of us was sure where we were headed. Through the mist we heard the commotion of another postrace party, which would last late into the night. I was the bowman for this race, the first to see how the entrance to the harbor broke hard to port, seemingly eager to eat its own tail. As the channel narrowed, I trained the beam of the Coleman flashlight on the red warning buoys for Dad, who was at the helm. He throttled back on the engine, and I felt the vibrations under my feet. Without much headway, we were taken hold of by the last of the big waves from the lake pitching our craft from side to side. We held on as we moved slowly ahead into the gloom. The channel continued to curve back on itself, and I swung the beam of light from one side to the other, looking for any sign of life.

Finally, we came around the final turn, and there in front of us lay the rest of the fleet, our competitors for the next day. The entire harbor was filled with boats. There were so many that one could cross from one side to the other by hopping from one vessel to the next until reaching land. We tied off to the end of this conga line, and some of the crew did step lively ashore for a drink or two or three. But Dad, Chris, and I stayed aboard, eating leftovers and gazing about us in silence, simply happy to have made it this far.

Years later, my mother-in-law lived a short walk from Bronte Harbor. As I said, we loved to visit for the Christmas holidays, and if the weather wasn't too cold we would take a stroll down to the pier and the nearby beach. In the dead of winter, with the leaves gone from the trees and a few inches of snow on the ground, the entranceway and docks appeared downright quaint, nothing to think twice about. Yet any sailor can tell you how quickly the forecast can change. How in short order the wind can begin to blow and the waves will build and build on themselves until this crossing becomes a white-knuckler.

24

Far beyond our world of the water, ball diamond, and ice rink, the campaign against cancer was reaching a fever pitch. A full-page advertisement ran in the *New York Times*, urging President Richard Nixon to become fully involved. "Mr. Nixon: You can cure cancer," it read.

Only a few years before, many couldn't bring themselves to say the word "cancer" aloud, as if doing so would invite an evil spirit into a home. Now stories about cancer seemed to be everywhere. The movie *Love Story* would be followed by *Brian's Song*, the true-life story of Brian Piccolo, Chicago Bears running back, and his battle against testicular cancer, and then *Bang the Drum Slowly*, about a ballplayer with Hodgkin's disease. Aleksandr Solzhenitsyn's *Cancer Ward*, an account of a cancer hospital in the Soviet Union, became a best seller, while op-ed columns and letters ran in newspapers across the country, often urging that more money be spent on cancer research. Now the words "cancer" and "cure" were being used together not only in publications like *Look* magazine but during congressional hearings as well.

Mary Lasker, a lobbyist, worked behind the scenes for the passage of a sweeping bill on Capitol Hill. She convinced her close friend Eppie Lederer (aka Ann Landers), who penned the popular advice column, to help her. On April 20, 1971, Landers told her readers that if they were looking for a laugh to turn the page, but if not, she asked, "If a country of ours can put a man on the moon why can't we find a cure for cancer?"

Landers echoed Lasker's approach that a cure for cancer needed political will as well as medical advances. In other words, if Washington could deliver the money, the doctors would do the rest. Landers told her readers to back Senate Bill S-34. "If enough citizens let their senators know they want Bill S-34 passed, it will pass."

The response was overwhelming, with cards and letters pouring into Capitol Hill. Missouri senator Stuart Symington urged Landers to call off the dogs. "Please, Eppie," he wrote her. "I got the message."

"Your brother was at Roswell Park during an exceptional time," Lucius Sinks pointed out to me when we got together again. "Real progress was being made on the medical front with the clinical trials and now there was more money for research. We were receiving sizeable funds from the State of New York, with Governor Nelson Rockefeller being in our corner, as well as state senator Earl Brydges. Never underestimate how much Senator Brydges helped out western New York. In addition, we had the grants from NCI. You could say that these were the halcyon days of Roswell Park."

"So what changed?"

Sinks smiled. "Sometimes you don't realize the impact of something until it is well played out," he said. "By 1971, events were building for more money from Washington. I mean millions and millions of dollars, which was a good thing, I suppose."

"But more money didn't cure all of cancer."

"No, it didn't," Sinks replied. "This is going to sound sort of counterintuitive, but more and more money doesn't always help."

"Why's that?"

"I've come to believe that progress was first made in leukemia because there wasn't a ton of money to be made in pediatrics back then," Sinks continued. "Any progress made at Roswell Park or elsewhere didn't cost the doctors already in the field. Few of them in pediatrics had any financial stake in what we were doing, so they weren't concerned about such changes."

"That meant you were left alone? To do your work?"

Sinks nodded. "We could keep looking for possible solutions. That only a few of us were in this area back then helped foster more cooperation."

"But when more money from D.C. entered the picture in 1971—"

"It was an impressive amount," Sinks said. Indeed, it was a total of $1.5 billion over three years. "I know people fought long and hard to bring that into the picture. You need every kind of resource you can find in going against this disease."

Sinks paused and then began again. "It may seem strange to say, but you have to remember money doesn't fix everything, certainly not overnight. You needed other factors to go in your favor too."

As we talked, it struck me that one needed to have a very particular, nuanced approach to do this kind of work. One in which bigger wasn't always better—a world in which more money didn't necessarily translate to better results.

"When a kid, a patient of yours, died?" I began.

"Yes?"

"Obviously, it had to be devastating."

"Sure it was. Some nurses and doctors talk about their angels," Sinks replied. "They're the patients that you'll never forget. The ones you tried so hard to save."

Many of the doctors in this field have an intimate relationship with death. Of course, Donald Pinkel came close to dying himself.

Jerry Yates lost one of his first patients to cancer. James Holland had patients, including T. J. Martell, whom he couldn't save. (Martell's father, Tony, was an executive in the music industry and started a foundation in his son's name.)

As Sinks and I discussed this, I had to ask him, "Do you think you see death differently than normal people? Than the rest of us?"

Sinks shrugged. "I don't know about that."

"But you've told me that you had patients pass away with you at their bedside. You've seen a lot more of death than most other people."

"True," Sinks said.

We had finished our lunches, and soon the waiter cleared the dishes. Around us, we had again outlasted another lunchtime crowd. After filling almost to capacity, the room was mostly empty as we finished our conversation.

I started again. "What you went through—doing the work you did—that must change a person, don't you think?"

"I suppose so," Sinks said. "But who's to say exactly how? All I know is that we had a job, a goal. Almost every day we felt like we were getting closer, that we could solve this riddle, really help more kids. Many of us—despite disagreements about a particular drug or treatment—many of us felt the same. So you learn to keep going."

"Regardless of how much grant money is coming in or the politics involved?"

"Regardless of how much money is out there," Sinks replied. "At least I did, so did Jim Holland and so did many of the others. To do this kind of work, you have to believe that the next answer is out there, what you need to know is around the next corner. You have to believe that if you keep going, you might just find it."

"Could this work, this kind of research, be done today?" I ask. "In our world of managed care?

Sinks smiled. "I don't know. I mean there's great work going in medicine right now, but ours was a different time. As you know, we were forced to do a lot of it ourselves."

"Holland learned about that enzyme from the pig liver," I said. "How he had to do it himself."

Sinks answered, "When it came right down to it we all had to do something like that for ourselves at some point. It forced us to really think about this disease and what it could do, what we could do. Maybe it forced us to become more involved than we ever planned to be."

When Sinks was the chief cancer research pediatrician at Roswell Park, Cyril Garvey, an attorney from Sharon, Pennsylvania, and his wife, Claudia, began to stay for extended periods in downtown Buffalo. Their son, Kevin, three years older than my brother, had become a patient at Roswell Park, suffering from acute leukemia. While the Garvey family could afford to stay in a local hotel, the father noticed people were sleeping in their cars outside the hospital. Cyril Garvey thought they were homeless. But when he was told those were the parents of other kids at Roswell Park, those who couldn't afford a room for the night, he was dumbfounded at first.

In January 1972, Kevin Garvey lost his battle with leukemia at the age of thirteen. Despite the loss, the Garvey family moved ahead with plans to help house families with children at Roswell Park and neighboring Buffalo General Hospital. Cyril Garvey joined with Rev. Edward Ulaszeski and Virginia Brady, the hospital director of social services, to purchase a three-story frame house at 782 Ellicott Street, one block away from Roswell Park. Throughout the spring and into the summer, a group of local volunteers refurbished it, and on July 26, 1972, the Kevin Guest House became the nation's first hospital hospitality facility, the forerunner of the Ronald McDonald House. In the years after that, additional buildings were purchased and renovated. Today, the complex has four apartments adjacent to the main building. One is completely handicapped accessible.

"Kevin Garvey is one of my patients that I'll never forget," Sinks said.

"Would you consider the Kevin Guest House to be part of your legacy there?" I asked.

"'Legacy' can be one of those fancy terms," the doctor replied. "I'm not sure what to make of such things."

"Well, let me rephrase it then. Is the Kevin Guest House, a facility that became a fixture at hospitals nationwide, among the things you're the most proud of during your time at Roswell Park? Something that you helped make a reality?"

Sinks smiled. "I like the phrasing of that a bit better."

"And is it?"

"It makes me feel good that it's been expanded several times— still going strong," he said. "I had a small part in getting it off the ground. It was one of many things we were trying to do and perhaps it was overlooked when it opened. But the Kevin Guest House became one of those hard-earned victories that one really treasures. Something you look back on years later and you realize how much good it did for so many families and so many kids."

25

About the time my brother was admitted to Roswell Park, James Holland began work on the germ-free units, the so-called Life Islands, at the hospital. Chemotherapy patients would reside for several weeks, even months, in this protected environment, until their bodies became strong enough to protect themselves against infection. As the new clinical trials stretched remission periods from weeks to months to years, the issue became, what could put the entire procedure over the top? What could keep patients healthy enough that the steady rounds of chemotherapy and other treatments could be stopped altogether?

The original isolator unit was simply a large plastic bubble inflated around a hospital bed, similar to what the actor John Travolta endured in the movie *The Boy in the Plastic Bubble* and what was reprised in a much more comic light by Jake Gyllenhaal in *Bubble Boy* twenty-five years later. But soon Holland upgraded to a larger setup that Jerry Yates explained was a germ-free room within a regular hospital room. The walls were made of plastic, and the patient could draw curtains for privacy. In addition to a bed, the germ-free unit had a table and chairs, telephone, and television. Purified air entered the room via a designated inlet, and any visitors were required to be dressed in sterilized spacesuits.

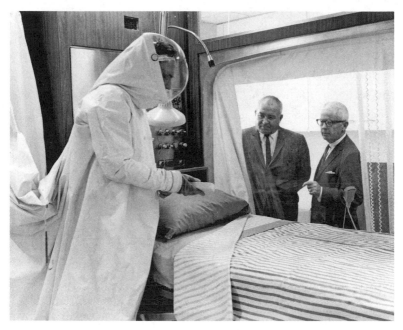

Courtesy of the Roswell Park Cancer Institute.

The germ-free units were on the third floor at Roswell Park, and they soon included two-patient bedrooms, where those recovering from leukemia were separated by a curtain. Yates was the supervising physician, and Audrey Tuttolomondo the head nurse.

"I had been head nurse on a floor at Buffalo General when Holland and Roswell Park got the federal grant for the germ-free unit," Tuttolomondo said. "In looking back on it, I was interested in a new challenge, starting something new. Also, I like working directly with doctors. They can be less picky than other nurses."

Over a three-year period, fifty-two patients would stay in one of the germ-free units. They ranged in age from seventeen to seventy-three years old. From the beginning, the biggest question was how well patients could tolerate being in isolation for perhaps weeks at a time. Even though all the patient beds were in view of the nurses' desk and telephones were in every unit, any objects entering the room, such as newspapers or books, needed to be sterilized. Food was passed into the units through a special door. It helped to have a sense of humor in such situations, and one patient, a seventeen-year-old, posted a sign that read, "Don't feed the animals."

Questions soon arose: Could the isolators help with younger patients like my brother? Keep them safe from infection as their immune systems recovered from the toxicity of the chemotherapy treatments? (Vince DeVita, who became the director of the National Cancer Institute, had a twelve-year-old son suffering from aplastic anemia, a condition in which the body stops producing enough blood cells. His son, Ted, was eventually housed in a sterile room at the NCI.)

In Buffalo, the doctors at Roswell Park initially held off because they were amazed by how quickly the younger leukemia patients rebounded. "[Children] are extremely resilient compared with adults," Yates said. "Unless they are severely ill, they are eating and playing normally even while getting chemotherapy. They don't seem to know how sick they are unless someone tells them. Keeping them in the real world was important because that facilitated their coping with the illness."

Also, Jimmie Holland soon noticed that something was missing with the older patients, the ones who lived for weeks at a time inside the isolator units. To make something come alive, all of the sensory details—sight, sound, smell, taste, and touch—need to be in play. Whether it's a book, movie, memory, or moment, these five elements often have to work in concert. Such components can elevate the everyday, even mundane, into something memorable, something to be treasured.

Patients in the isolation units were instructed to keep a diary, either in written entries or on tape recordings. On the third and twenty-first days in the unit, patients answered a questionnaire that often asked them to select the statement that "most nearly describes your own feelings."

In addition, nurses filled out questionnaires about the patients at the end of their eight-hour shifts. A fifty-one-item checklist tracked such topics as behavior, anxiety, and discomfort on a five-point scale. In looking at the responses by patients and nurses, as well as interviews with several of the doctors, Jimmie Holland determined that the patients, and even many of the nurses, missed the simple act of touch. As early as the third day inside the isolator, one-third of the patients said they missed this aspect of care the most.

One patient wrote, "The lack of direct touch and contact with people you love has created disturbances."

Another said, "You just feel you are all alone in the world and everything is cold and there is no warmth."

The rest of the senses "were adequately stimulated," Jimmie Holland wrote in a report about the germ-free unit. "Patients were not bored in general. . . . [But] the unexpected and frequently expressed loss was human touch."

Of the fifty-two patients who lived in the germ-free unit for several weeks, fifteen had complete remissions and five had partial remissions. Twelve experienced no remission, and twenty died while in the germ-free unit. In a subsequent report, Yates stated that the "failures to improve remission rate in patients with acute leukemia despite a reduction of infection has been disappointing." That left the doctors in Buffalo still searching for a procedure, treatment, or particular medicine that would make remission more permanent, especially with their younger patients. Once again they were reminded they were working far out on the fringe of the known world.

26

On this summer afternoon, Dad was constructing a clothes-line for Mom to hang the clean laundry. For the son of a civil engineer, such projects took on the gravitas of building the pyramids, and for this one, he decided that the anchoring posts would be placed several feet into the ground. For much of the morning, he dug two holes before preparing to mix the concrete base.

"Now you kids stay out of that hole," Dad told us. "I'll be right back with the Sakrete."

He dumped the last of the dirt out along the property line and pushed the wheelbarrow back to the garage. He moved at a good clip because he didn't trust us. And he had good reason.

Part of growing up in a large family is the pranks, teasing, ribbing, and general cruelty that goes into the dynamics between siblings. As soon as Dad was out of view, Susan began to talk to Chris, who was then the youngest.

"Don't you want to see what it's like to be down in that hole?" she asked him.

Chris, to his credit, shook his head.

"You can hop down in there for a minute," she continued. "Just a little while and then Tim and I will help you out. Won't we, Tim?"

I nodded dutifully, willing to be a part of my sister's schemes. Chris stayed rooted, glancing from her to the hole in front of us.

"C'mon, you can tell us all about it," Susan said. "Hop in and we'll pull you out."

"You promise?"

"Cross my heart and hope to die," his big sister answered. "And Tim does too, right?"

I shrugged, curious about how this would play out.

Chris edged closer to the hole, and Susan came alongside him. For a moment, I thought she was going to give him a little nudge. But she only watched as he squatted down and then slid off the edge, into the hole. As with many things like this, once a person falls into the situation, it can be deeper, more overwhelming than he ever thought it would be.

"Now get me out," Chris said. His chin perhaps came up to the level of the ground. He put his hands up on the edge, trying to pull himself back to level ground. But it was no use. "Time to get me out," he repeated. "You promised."

Yet Susan was already walking away. Down in the garage, we heard Dad rummaging around, readying the concrete mix.

"He'll be back soon," Susan told me. "And he'll be plenty mad."

That's how both of us ended up walking away, leaving Chris in the hole.

Of course, Dad was plenty mad when he returned. First he yelled at Chris, telling him never to trust his siblings again. Later, when he had calmed down, he met with me, asking why we had done it, why we had disobeyed his orders. An Old Testament father would have given me a tongue-lashing or much worse. But, if anything, Dad was more curious about why we had done such a thing. Why had we left our little brother stranded in a hole in the backyard?

"You have to be better to people, especially your family, than that," he said. "You don't have to like them, you don't have to always get along, but you have to stick by them."

During Eric's illness, we became much better at hanging together, looking out for each other. By this point, my brother's maintenance program was supplemented by injections of methotrexate into the spinal cord every few weeks. These started after another test showed a brief spike in pressure inside the skull, perhaps a rise in the cerebrospinal fluid. That could have been a sign that the cancer had found refuge in the brain and the spine. Yet as quickly as such symptoms were detected, they somehow disappeared. More extensive examinations were scheduled, including a retest of the Salk vaccine, but nothing out of the ordinary revealed itself. During this period, Eric's appetite increased and he gained 15 to 20 pounds, which the doctors saw as a good development.

A physical examination "revealed a well-developed and well-nourished child, who appears to be in no distress," one examining doctor wrote.

"Physical exam is essentially within normal limits," another wrote a few months later.

". . . is essentially within normal limits," another doctor repeated four weeks later.

While my brother remained in remission, nobody, including his doctors, could say with any certainty how long he would remain there. That said, Eric had technically been in remission since early October 1967—thirty-eight months and counting. This was a miraculous turnaround for a kid who was supposed to live no more than eighteen months when he was first diagnosed with ALL. The nationwide effort against cancer, at least against childhood leukemia, was being won right before our eyes.

On the home front, we proved to be a resilient crew. By this point, with Mom up at Roswell Park on a regular basis, the freezer was filled with casseroles that we reheated in her absence. We all had our tasks and duties. I secured my driver's permit at the earliest opportunity and then took a driver's ed class so I could chauffeur my siblings without any restrictions. With my grandmother's guidance, Susan became a respectable chef, ready to cook the next family dinner, if need be. Middle brother Chris babysat the little ones, leading them on scavenger hunts and games of hide-and-seek. It was his idea to bring in guinea pigs and hamsters and to put together a small aquarium that Eric, especially, loved. Of course, we always had dogs in our family—a parade of Irish setters and, later on, golden retrievers. Whether this was by design or accident didn't matter. For as Milan Kundera wrote, "Dogs are our link to paradise. They don't know evil or jealousy or discontent. To sit with a dog on a hillside on a glorious afternoon is to be back in Eden, where doing nothing was not boring—it was peace."

Most families have one big brother or big sister. From an age standpoint, I was that designee in my family, and to this day the title that perhaps I'm the most proud of is being the oldest of six kids. Yet the only way any of this worked for as long as it did is that we had several big brothers. There were many roles to fill and tasks to do, which would have been daunting if we looked too far into the future. Without realizing it, we had learned to stay in the present. It didn't matter if we were on the boat or not; we had learned enough to read the winds of circumstance and adjust the sails accordingly. Somehow we did what needed to be done, day after day, crossing after crossing.

Decades later, my sister Susan visited the Freer Gallery of Art, which borders the National Mall in Washington, D.C. There she

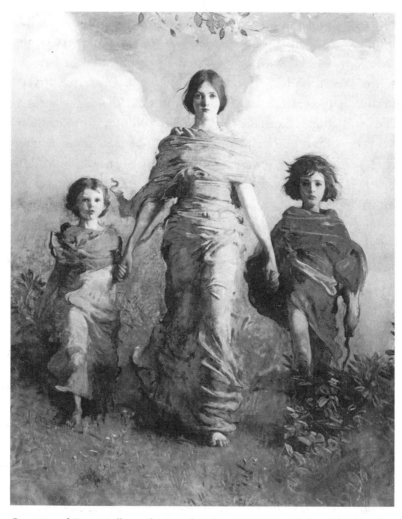

Courtesy of Freer Gallery of Art and Arthur M. Sackler Gallery, Smithsonian Institution, Washington, D.C. Gift of Charles Lang Freer, F1893.11a.

came face to face with a striking painting by Abbott Handerson Thayer entitled *A Virgin*. In it a robed young woman holds the hand of a younger girl and wild-haired boy, and three abreast they stride toward the viewer.

"This is how I think of those times when we were left in charge of what was left of the family," she said. "I saw the Thayer painting in the stairwell in the Freer and it just knocked me over, bringing me back to being fifteen years old and having it be my responsibility to care for Chris, Bryan, and Amy so much of the time."

One night, with Mom and Dad at Roswell Park, Susan decided that the occasion required "something noteworthy," and she proceeded to give Chris, Bryan, and Amy haircuts. First she washed their hair in the bathroom sink and then carefully trimmed their bangs and pruned the tops and the sides as best she could.

"I was pretty proud of myself," she said, "but Mom and Dad, if they did come home from the hospital that night, were too tired to notice."

For the Thanksgiving holiday, we always played touch football at our house or, better yet, up in Lockport in the park across the street from the hospital where Eric had first been diagnosed, which housed the children's wing where they didn't know what to do with him. The Turkey Bowl drew a good crowd, with several of my friends dropping by. What gave some of them pause was how the steroid intake, the combination of meds, had caused Eric to put on so much weight, even swelling his face.

"He's the husky Wendel," somebody said, and that afternoon he was nicknamed "Beefy" and "Porky."

I should have stepped in—told everyone to stop it, just shut up. But Eric shot me a look, urging me to be quiet. That day he was interested only in playing football. If anything, he seemed concerned that any disagreement would break up the game. So we played on under gray skies, with the promise of snow.

Perhaps it was the cold weather, or the growing number of players, but the game soon became chippy. Instead of two hands touch above the waist, the ball carrier was routinely sent flying with an extra hard push. Blocks along the line took on an extra vengeance.

Usually touch football becomes a passing game, stressing how well the quarterback can throw and his receivers can catch. But in the swirling winds and cold, nobody could hang on to the slick ball very well. As a result, my team stopped throwing the ball all together. As the quarterback and play-caller, I couldn't grip the pigskin and as a lark I handed the ball off to Eric, who ran with choppy, determined steps right up the middle, sending bodies flying.

"Same play," I said in the huddle. Once again I stepped back to pass, only to hand the ball off to Eric, who put his head down and ran straight ahead.

"What have you been putting in his feed?" somebody on the other team cried out. "Spinach?"

"Wonder drugs," somebody else said.

We ran the same play again: Eric lugging the ball with both hands up the middle. Though it wasn't hard to touch him, nobody on the other team wanted to get that close to my little brother. Trying to stop him took a piece out of you. Guys on the other team fell to the ground, mud smearing their jeans and sweatshirts.

"Again?" I asked Eric in the huddle. He only smiled and nodded.

We continued to run variations of the same play—Eric straight up the gut, Eric around either end—and we soon scored.

As I watched my brother roll into the end zone, covered in muck and with a huge grin on his face, I realized that he had become tougher than the rest of us. He didn't care about the teasing, the lousy weather, or the wet field. Right before our eyes, he had risen above it all. We were afraid of such things, the pain that could be upon us, that could overwhelm us. Eric had moved past such concerns long ago.

27

On October 11, 1971, the Subcommittee of Public Health and the Environment of the House and Foreign Commerce Committee held hearings at Roswell Park in Buffalo. Several of the ALGB leukemia doctors testified at this session and other hearings in the months leading up to possible action on Capitol Hill. None was more determined to see such landmark legislation reach the president's desk for his signature than James Holland.

"I believe there has been a broad and powerful wave of advances in cancer research . . . ," he told the congressional group. "In some places, the tide has raced ahead, providing enough knowledge for prevention or cure. When applied in those places, prevention and cure has resulted. The value of such observations is clear. We know it can be done, because it has been done. . . . I believe a greater effort can and should be sustained, one that can and should be successful."

Even with momentum building in Congress and in the White House for a $1.5 billion program to battle cancer, not everyone in the medical community shared Holland's optimism or fervor for action.

"We must not be guilty of 'overpromise' to the American people," said Dr. John Hogness, president of the Institute of Medicine of the National Academy of Sciences. "We have come far in our understanding of the basic processes that occur in malignant disease, but we are certainly not on the threshold of a breakthrough that suddenly will reduce cancer to as minor a health problem as, for example, smallpox has become."

Dr. John A. D. Cooper, president of the Association of American Medical Colleges, reminded everyone that, despite recent progress, "the fundamental fact remains—the basic causes and nature of the cancerous process are unknown. The nature of cancer is deeply embedded in the most elemental life processes and is an obscure and complex part of the life cycle."

Despite such divisions, the American Cancer Society strongly backed the federal legislation. Dr. H. Marvin Pollard, the ACS president, called the "abrupt response of many distinguished scientists that we do not know enough about cancer to mount a more dynamic, massive effort against this disease through a new administrative design is perhaps an indirect recognition that individually, as basic scientists in fields other than cancer, they honestly do not know enough about cancer. This is understandable. But we in the cancer field disagree with these men, many of whom are esteemed colleagues; they are men of integrity, but in this case their judgment is wrong."

Despite opposition, the measure passed on Capitol Hill, and on December 23, 1971, at noon in the State Dining Room at the White House, President Richard Nixon signed the National Cancer Act. The legislation had seen swift passage in the Senate, thanks to the bipartisan support of Edward Kennedy (D-MA) and Jacob Javits (R-NY), only to stall in the House of Representatives.

Nixon had an eye on reelection the following year and pushed hard for this measure, which many believed could be a part of his presidential legacy. As the *Chicago Tribune* noted, if the president could put "an end to the war in Vietnam and defeat the ravages of cancer—then he will have carved himself in the history of this nation a niche of Lincolnesque proportions, for he will have done more than put a man on the moon."

Thanks to pressure from the White House, as well as the public campaign by Mary Lasker, the effort's chief lobbyist, a modified version eventually passed the House and was sent to the president to sign. Sitting behind a small wooden desk, Nixon told the overflow crowd before signing the bill, "I hope that in the years ahead that we may look back on this day and this action as being the most significant action taken during my administration."

The president noted that many in attendance had never witnessed a signing at the White House. "I will use two pens for the signature," he told them, "but a souvenir pen will be available to everybody in the audience here. We had to stretch a little to find that many, but we did it."

With Nixon's signature, the "War on Cancer" had a new infusion of serious cash. A total of $1.5 billion was targeted to be spent over the next three years—$400 million for 1972, $500 million for 1973, and $600 million for 1974.

In addition, the new program stated that the number of cancer research institutes would be increased to fifteen nationwide and that these locations would be eligible to receive grants up to $5 million annually. The new legislation also called for the establishment of a cancer research program within the National Cancer Institute. The budget for this new program, which was intended to coordinate and intensify efforts to find a cure for cancer, would be sent directly to the president, with the secretary of Health and Human Services, the director of the National Institutes of Health (NIH), and the National Cancer Advisory Board instructed to comment on but not change the bottom line. After being outside the medical mainstream, often ostracized by their peers, the leukemia doctors now found themselves front and center. The National Cancer Act brought in not only a huge infusion of money but plenty of other institutions and hospitals.

With a stroke of the presidential pen, the leukemia doctors' "fiercest critics were supposed to now be with us," Lucius Sinks said. "One big cooperative group."

It wouldn't quite work out that way.

28

When Eric relapsed for the penultimate time, he was given a combination of vincristine and prednisone, which once again stabilized him. After that, the doctors at Roswell Park put him on two new drugs. One was l-asparaginase, or asparaginase, which targeted a chemical that both normal cells and cancer cells need to survive. The goal was to kill the cells that were rapidly dividing, but as with many chemotherapy treatments, the drugs couldn't tell the difference between cancerous cells and normal cells. The second new drug was Cytoxan, another derivative of mustard gas that had proven effective against a wide range of cancers. The side effects included low blood cell counts and an increased risk for anemia and infection.

The use of these two drugs underscored the growing concern about leukemia cells finding shelter in the central nervous system. After Donald Pinkel's success in Memphis, more hospitals, including Roswell Park for a time, turned to using varying programs of radiation treatments as well. But had they arrived at the point where treatment was too costly for the patients' long-term well-being? As Tom Junod wrote in *Esquire* decades later, "Radiation inflames, radiation scars, radiation creates adhesions, radiation damages nerves and blood vessels. . . . Worst of all, it's irreversible."

In August 1972, my brother was given a treatment of 2,400 rads of radiation to the skull. (A "significant amount," an expert told me.) Later studies revealed that children who were given such dosages repeatedly saw their IQ drop by 15 points or more.

"Every time I took Eric to Roswell Park, we were never sure if we'd be going home that day or be there for a week or more," Mom said. "It was like that with the radiation. When they told me that they were going to do it, I knew that this was their best guess about what was needed right now. I never argued with any of it."

When I asked Lucius Sinks about such procedures, he put me in touch with Cheryl Tabone, who still lives in the Buffalo suburbs. Her daughter, Angelique, is in her mid-forties and now cancer free. But over the previous twenty years, she has had surgery for brain tumors and lost the hearing in one ear. Angelique's IQ dropped, and her mother believes she is at a higher risk for dementia as she grows older.

"When you're putting a patient, beginning as a toddler, through these kinds of treatments, it has an effect," Cheryl Tabone said. "It becomes a big part of her life."

Angelique lives with her parents and finds it difficult to hold down a job. She worked at a childcare center for a few years and at the Wegmans supermarket near their home in Williamsville, New York. She was in the bakery for a time and then helping customers in the upstairs café. Her mother says that the management at Wegmans tried to find a place for her daughter, but it didn't work out.

"Do I blame the doctors for everything that she went through with the leukemia? No, I don't," Cheryl Tabone said. "The chemo, even the two weeks of radiation she had—that's all they had to work with back then. They did their best with what they had— what they understood at the time."

Throughout this period, the doctors tried various approaches to prevent the leukemia cells from settling in the central nervous system without deploying cranial irradiation. Pharmacological data showed that methotrexate, the chemotherapy drug that dated back to the 1950s, might be effective, and it was once again called to the forefront. The new approach called for it to be injected intrathecally (directly into the spinal canal) to stymie any meningeal relapse. This time, Dr. Arnold Freeman at Roswell Park, with input from Sinks and Holland, decided to change how it was used. Instead of high doses for concentrated periods of time, Freeman opted for lower amounts of methotrexate deployed over longer, more extended periods of time. Freeman wrote that this approach might be "capable of diffusing across the central nervous system barrier in amounts adequate to eradicate the leukemic cells."

Promising preliminary results soon led to a larger, randomized clinical trial, No. 7611. The study enrolled 634 patients, all of whom were younger than twenty years old. Treatment assignments were given out in sealed envelopes, with all the patients starting off with the familiar combination of vincristine and prednisone. More than 90 percent of the patients went into remission. Once again, the key became how best to keep them there. One group received radiation to the entire brain down to the second vertebra of the spinal column for a period of sixteen days; both eyes were shielded during such treatments. Methotrexate was also used.

The second group didn't receive any radiation. Instead an "intermediate dose" of methotrexate, correlated to the patient's weight, was given three times at three-week intervals. One-third of the dose was given in a concentrated amount, with the majority allowed to flow intravenously over a twenty-four-hour period. Additional rounds of methotrexate were given via spinal injections, and patients were required to stay well hydrated.

In further treatments developed at Roswell Park, patients were also given a reduced folic acid, usually administered as a short burst in the child's IV. Doctors characterized it as a "rescue agent" for the patient's normal cells.

Overall, the new approaches worked well, with 94 percent of the patients able to tolerate the full regimen. The toxicity of the intermediate dose of methotrexate "was within acceptable limits," Freeman wrote in the *New England Journal of Medicine.*

29

Even though we regularly listened to the weather forecasts out of Buffalo and Toronto before we sailed the inland sea, rarely did the predictions play out exactly as planned. Once we went down to the boat and Dad told everyone to bring aboard a jacket or a sweatshirt. Winds were forecast to be strong out of the west. Certainly everyone at Olcott Yacht Club had gotten the word for we were the only boat heading out of the harbor early that Saturday morning.

Still, once we were a few miles offshore, what wind there was soon slackened, and our progress slowed to next to nothing. I brought up a packet of crackers from the galley, and we munched them in boredom.

"Are we in the doldrums?" Chris asked.

"Where'd you hear about the doldrums?" Susan asked.

"In social studies class. We talked about how the wind would disappear for so long that they had to throw their horses overboard, so the top of the sails could catch any breeze."

"Sounds like they were dum-dums," Eric chimed in.

We gazed about us at the glassy surface of the big lake.

"Anything could beat us right now," Susan said. "Even a cracker." With that, she flipped her saltine over the side.

We watched as it bobbed along in the water, slowly edging away and now seemingly moving ahead of us.

"We're getting beat by a cracker," Bryan said.

"Getting beat pretty bad too," Eric added.

With nothing better to do, we watched as the cracker seemed to pick up speed, floating away from us, bound for the far horizon.

Out in the middle of the lake sometimes all we could do was blink our eyes in disbelief. Dad talked about how lines of mountains or what looked like stands of Christmas trees sometimes seemed to come into view on the far horizon when a cold front was approaching, caused by the sudden change in temperature. Old-timers down at the Olcott Yacht Club talked about how pillars of mist, resembling so many campfires, could rise into the sky on December days when winter's first ice formed along the shoreline.

Ontario, perhaps more than any other Great Lake, laid claim to a long gauntlet of unusual phenomena. Waterspouts were blamed for the sinking of a number of ships, including the paddle wheelers *Princess Charlotte, Homer Warren, Rambler, Blackbird,* and *Farmer's Daughter.* Sometimes when the water surface was as smooth as glass and the wind died down to nothing, it was as if the sides of the lake decided to move in closer so that everyone could have a better look. In scientific terms, this was called refraction. Yet simple scientific definitions couldn't take away the wonder of seeing trees and buildings, even smoke from a distant lake freighter, come into view with vivid detail and clarity.

Such sightings dated back to the early days on the Great Lakes. In August 1856, the *Lockport Journal* wrote about how passengers on the steamer *Bay State* were treated to a splendid mirage, a classic case of refraction, on another trip across Lake Ontario.

"It occurred just as the sun was setting, at which time some 12 vessels were seen on the horizon, in an inverted position, with a distinctness and vividness truly surprising," the dispatch read. "The atmosphere was overcast with a thick haze such as precedes a storm, and of a color favorable to represent upon the darkened background, vividly, the full outlines of the rigging, sails, etc., as perfect as if the ships themselves were actually transformed to the aerial canvas. The unusual phenomenon lasted until darkness put an end to the show."

One didn't necessarily need to be on the water to witness such apparitions. Once my brother Chris and I were walking on the stone beach down by the Olcott piers, an hour or so before sunset, when on the far horizon the new spires of Toronto somehow could be seen in rich detail, hovering above the horizon line. We gazed at the glorious sight, so clear for a moment that we could see traffic lights on city streets many miles away. We watched transfixed, like passengers on the *Bay State*, until the sun set.

When the cracker disappeared from view, all of us found a place to hunker down. Susan was already reading in the shade of the foredeck. Sometimes she would read aloud to the younger kids, but nobody was interested this afternoon. We could have been back on shore, playing ball up on the West Bluff. At times like these, I never understood what we were doing out on the lake, wasting another summer day when there had to be better things going on back on dry land.

I stretched out on the foredeck, looking up at the blue sky. This part of the boat became the domain of us older kids, with the younger ones in orange life jackets staying down in the cockpit. Chris retrieved a transistor radio from down below and tuned in some music.

A few weeks before, I had been at Burg's family cottage after dinner, waiting until the last minute before biking back down to our place on Van Buren Street. We were all getting into music back then, and Sharon, Burg's older sister, let us borrow some of her records—the Beatles and the like. All of us had saved up for small transistor radios, and one night after playing ball on the West Bluff, we were sitting around the long table in the Buergers' sunroom when Danny Stein pulled open the back door with a wild look on his face. He had been riding his bike from his parents' cottage, a quarter mile or so to the west.

"I dropped my radio," he said.

"You break it?" Burg asked.

"No, but check this out," he said, holding up the small GE model. He turned up the volume, and at first all we heard was static. "It's better out here," he said, waving us toward the door, "closer to the lake."

In the dark, we followed him through the Buergers' backyard to the wooden stairs that led down to a stone wall at the water's edge. With each step, the signal became stronger, and we drew closer, listening to Danny's radio. A smattering of music, an upbeat lead-in, was followed by an announcer welcoming us back to "WJR and our coverage of this year's Michigan State Fair."

"You've got Detroit," Burg said.

"Must be the conditions tonight," Danny said, gazing up at the cloudless sky and wide swath of stars.

"So if you can bring in Detroit, what else can you get?"

Slowly Danny inched the dial along with his thumb, trolling past snippets and static, until we were listening to a baseball game. At first, we had no idea where it was from and didn't recognize any of the names. At Burg's we regularly played All-Time, All-Star Baseball, a board game put out by *Sports Illustrated* magazine. That had gotten us up to speed on many of the stars of yesteryear—Joe DiMaggio, Satchel Paige, Chief Bender, Home Run Baker, and Mordecai Brown. We loved the names as much as the games themselves, playing several rounds every night after sunset. Such make-believe contests afforded us the chance to assemble all-star teams going back through the years for the Yankees, Athletics, Red Sox, and Dodgers. We played so often that summer we wore the numbers right off the dice and had to write new numbers on with white hockey tape.

But that was all in the world of Olcott, and so much of it was in our heads. Here was a live game that wasn't the hometown Buffalo Bisons or anything else nearby. We listened in silence until the end of the inning and the station identification.

"We'll be back after this commercial break," we were told. "You're listening to KMOX radio, the flagship station of the St. Louis Cardinals."

"St. Louis?" Burg said. "You've pulled in St. Louis."

"I don't know how," Danny said, staring back up at the sky, as if it was some kind of visitation from the far side of the world.

And there we sat, together on the stairs leading down to the lake, listening to big-league action from a bona fide ballpark, enjoying another of Lake Ontario's mirages.

The afternoon of the cracker and being in the doldrums, Chris easily found WKBW out of Buffalo. It was one of the local stations we could always pull in. We listened to the Rascals singing about "People Got to Be Free," followed by Gary Puckett's "Young Girl." This wouldn't last for long. Dad didn't appreciate such music. He still pined for the days of folk music, when Joan Baez; Peter, Paul, and Mary; and Bob Dylan (before he went electric) could be found on the radio. After another song or two, he would invariably tell Chris to "turn off that racket," and the radio would be stowed back down below.

High above me, I heard the main halyard slap once, then twice against the 30-foot aluminum mast. This time we wouldn't have to worry about rock-and-roll music igniting another family argument. As Tommy James and the Shondells began to sing, "Mony, Mony," I glanced off to the west. Far away, the water surface had already been transformed from a glassy sheen to dimples and now rough edges due to the weather front already bearing down on us.

"Here it comes," I said, heading down to the cockpit.

Above us, the weather vane at the top of the mast swung around, now pointing due west. The wind continued to gust, funneling right down the lake.

Those initial gusts caused us to heel over to the starboard side, and Dad expertly let out the mainsail. I took the helm as Susan and Chris trimmed the sails.

For a moment, Dad just stood there, his face breaking into a big grin. "I told you we'd have some wind today," he nodded at Mom. "It just took it a little while to find us."

30

After graduating from Niagara University Nursing School, Catherine Lyons planned to work at Buffalo Children's Hospital in labor and delivery. Bringing newborns into the world sounded like the most fun a person new to medicine could have.

To guarantee that she got a job, Lyons also interviewed at Roswell Park, and "at first I just hated it," she said. In the early 1970s, the hospital was known as an aging physical plant where too many of its patients died. Yet when Lyons began to talk with the staff, especially the nurses, she met "a group of people who weren't interested in doing something that was easy. They chose something that was hard and found the satisfaction and reward in that."

Lyons took a job at Roswell Park and planned to stay a year, until something at Buffalo Children's or elsewhere opened up. Instead, she was there for nearly a quarter century and rose to become chief nursing officer.

Many of the nurses at Roswell Park had been on their way to someplace else, with other goals in mind, when they arrived in Buffalo. While the work could be demanding and the hours long, at Roswell Park they often found themselves on par with the doctors. They attended many of the same meetings, sitting at the same table where major decisions about pending treatments and clinical trials were made. At Roswell Park, they discovered that their opinions mattered.

"Our nurses were right there with us on the front lines," James Holland said. "They were with the patients on a daily basis more than us. We would have been fools not to listen to what they had to say. They knew what we were up against better than anybody else."

Brenda Hall went to Sweet Home High School in suburban Buffalo and attended college at Utica State. She almost quit after her first few days in pediatrics at Roswell Park. One of the children she cared for, a young boy named John, died when she wasn't at the hospital, and the mother told her that one of the last things he did was ask for Hall.

"It was draining," she recalled. "Everyone had times where you wondered what you had gotten yourself into, how you're supposed to really do your job."

Sometimes a nurse's job became more difficult due to the patient's family. During my brother's time on 5E, other kids regularly called home, pleading with their parents to visit them. One father, a dapper-dressed local businessman, buttonholed one of the doctors, asking him, "When do you think my son is going to die?"

The doctor looked at him in disbelief.

"It would really help my schedule to know that," the father continued. "Surely, you have some idea."

"I don't know," the doctor snapped. "I'm not God."

As soon as Hall settled into her new job at Roswell Park, Lucius Sinks and other doctors told her to continue her medical training; treatments and procedures were changing in a hurry. As a result, she became one of the first nurse practitioners at the hospital. Hall said the nurses were urged to become experts in particular treatments and procedures. Okie Ok, for example, was known for finding veins, slowly rubbing the skin so another thin ribbon could rise to the surface after other veins had been depleted by frequent injections.

My brother's favorite was Diana Perry, an occupational therapist. Born and raised in Buffalo, she collected salt and pepper shakers, and marveled at the distances people came for treatment at Roswell Park. "We must be doing right here," she once told my mother, "because so many people come from miles around to get here."

Perry thought that Lockport was far away, and places like Albany and Pittsburgh might as well have been on the far side of the moon. She was happy riding the bus down Main Street to work, often bringing crayons and colored paper for the patients on 5E.

"She got their minds off their treatments," Hall said. "The kids just adored her."

31

The National Hockey League held its annual amateur draft on June 6, 1972, at the Queen Elizabeth Hotel in Montreal. It would be the longest draft to that point in hockey history, lasting almost four hours, and one of the most successful of all time. Future Hall of Famers Steve Shutt and Bill Barber as well as four future All-Stars were selected in the opening round, which saw the New York Islanders take Billy Harris with the first pick. Our Buffalo Sabres opted for Jim Schoenfeld, a rugged defenseman with the Niagara Falls Flyers, and he made the big-league team coming out of training camp.

At Roswell Park, Eric showed no ill effects from the radiation treatment or the heightened drug routine. A recent checkup noted that he "has been skating lately." In fact, Eric was back in uniform at the Kenan Center and avidly following Schoenfeld's rookie year with the Buffalo Sabres. The tall redhead had not only made the team but was on the top defense pairing, teamed with veteran Tim Horton. Thanks to an improved defense, the Sabres were on their way to the third-best single-season improvement to that point in the National Hockey League. In its third year of existence, the hometown team would reach the playoffs.

Throughout Eric's short life, my parents had decided time and again that they wouldn't overly protect him from the daily routine of life. My parents' definition of "normal" meant being involved in the day to day, playing on the local team, and going to school as many days as possible.

"We had decided that we weren't going to put him up on a shelf and say, 'Isn't he beautiful?'" Mom later told me. "Remember, your brother existed in two worlds—what we had at home and what was up at Roswell. The only thing he wanted was to be a part of both of them."

Soon after Thanksgiving, the first cases of chicken pox began to surface at Gasport Elementary School. Principal Fred Gibbs called Mom at home, and she notified the doctors in Buffalo. Several of us older kids had already had chicken pox, and my parents hoped Eric wouldn't contract it. But soon spots began to break out on his face and arms, and he needed to stay at home for at least a week so he wouldn't infect the other children at Roswell Park. For the next few days, Mom had Eric soak in the bathtub, and after he dried off, she covered the spots with pink calamine lotion.

"Today we know so much more about highly contagious viral infections," Donald Pinkel said. "How devastating it can be to a child whose immune system has been severely compromised by years of chemotherapy. We didn't know nearly enough to fully protect kids back then."

I wondered if Eric would have been a candidate for one of Roswell Park's "Life Islands" if the setting and technology had been better suited for younger patients.

"Possibly," Pinkel said. "But that and other procedures weren't ready yet. We were understanding more and more about disease. The question was, 'Could we do enough in the time we had to save more kids?' It was so much about time and the circumstances we were presented with. There were no easy answers to the questions we were all facing back then."

As our phone conversation came to an end, Pinkel asked for my home address, and a few days later a small manila envelope from him arrived. It was a study entitled "Chickenpox and Leukemia." He was the only author, and it had been printed in the *Journal of Pediatrics* in May 1961, before he left Roswell Park to build St. Jude Children's Research Hospital in Memphis. It detailed four case studies, four young leukemia patients who contracted chicken pox.

In the summary Pinkel wrote, "The serious nature of chickenpox complicating acute leukemia may be due to the leukemia itself or the drugs used to treat it. Adrenal steroids, 6-MP and Methotrexate all tend to inhibit immune response in certain situations." Farther down he wrote, "Exposure of susceptible children with leukemia to chickenpox should be avoided. When exposure or illness does occur, the physician should try to discontinue or reduce antileukemia chemotherapy if it seems feasible."

On a last page, Pinkel had attached a handwritten note with Scotch tape: "Subsequently varicella-zoster immune globulin (VZ1A) was developed and has been highly successful in prevention of V-Z in immunosuppressed patients of all types."

The chicken pox vaccine wasn't licensed for use until 1995. As a result, what was an innocent nuisance for most children, a rite of passage for many of us, carried a far greater risk for children with leukemia for many decades.

On December 5, 1972, Eric suffered "a complete relapse," according to Dr. J. J. Wang, who first examined him in Buffalo. His temperature soared, and he was severely fatigued. Here Eric's outpatient record shifts from typed lines, sometimes as many as a dozen or more at a time, to short handwritten sentences from the examining physicians. Eric was readmitted immediately to Roswell Park under Dr. Sinks's care; the old standbys, vincristine and prednisone, as well as methotrexate and 6-MP, were deployed. On the wall above his bed, Mom scotch-taped a black-and-white photo of Jim Schoenfeld.

Eight days after Eric relapsed, his hockey hero was caught up in the most memorable fight that ever occurred at War Memorial Auditorium in downtown Buffalo. The Boston Bruins, nicknamed the "Big, Bad Bruins," were in town and eager to put the upstart Sabres in their place.

Early in the first period, Schoenfeld checked Wayne Cashman, the Bruins' forward, into the far-end boards. The doors through which the Zamboni came in to resurface the ice hadn't been properly secured, and both players went sailing into the tunnel near the stands. Cashman came up swinging, and Schoenfeld returned the favor, catching the Bruin with a right cross. After Cashman landed a few punches, Schoenfeld neutralized him with a headlock as the linesman tried to step in. But the Buffalo rookie refused to let go, hitting Cashman several more times, bloodying his nose. By the time the evening ended, Schoenfeld would be in a total of three fights—the one with Cashman; a lopsided tilt over Carl Vadnais, rival defenseman; and a closer bout with Bobby Orr, the future Hall of Famer.

My brother didn't watch or hear the game. But he heard the nurses talking about it the next morning, about how Schoenfeld had single-handedly taken on the defending Stanley Cup champions.

The Christmas holidays arrived, and much of the Roswell Park staff, and any patient healthy enough, cleared out for a day or two. Only a skeleton crew remained, and on Christmas Eve, with the rest of us at home, Mom found an abandoned wheelchair.

"Hop in," she told her son. "It's time we cased this joint." As the snow fell outside, she wheeled him toward the elevators.

From a design standpoint, the old Roswell Park Memorial Institute building could be viewed as a cul-de-sac, vertically and horizontally. A hallway ran in a long line from the small street entrance to a series of five floors that were built one on top of another, forming what looked like a reverse letter C from on high. The top floor was the pediatrics, or children's, ward, an area isolated from the rest of the hospital.

The elevator doors opened, and Mom wheeled Eric inside. Together they rode down to the first floor and headed for the duck pond that stood in the lobby. The pond was home to several birds with clipped wings, and the ducks occasionally made a break for it, heading down the hallway of the first floor for the main entrance. At such times, the nurses were required to herd them back to the small pond.

A trio of ducks was quiet on this night, and Eric and Mom watched them for a time before returning to the elevator. On the second floor, they passed several administrative offices until they came to the Cigarette Hall of Fame, rolling past the eight-by-ten promotional shots of the celebrities, with Mom lingering in front of the photograph of Nat "King" Cole.

We have come a long way in how we view cancer, at least being able to call it by name today instead of the "C-word." Still, families often remain reluctant to publicize the specific kind of cancer a loved one suffered. As I said, I don't remember ever discussing leukemia as a family around the dinner table. Time and again, we were reminded that cancer could be the ultimate bogeyman, at least in our part of the world. We kids talked among ourselves, especially if Eric had to stay overnight at Roswell Park. We wondered when he could come back home. When Eric was first diagnosed, the cleaning lady who came in once a month abruptly quit. She became convinced that the disease was contagious and would infect her young son, too.

Today, we would like to think we have a better handle on such health issues. That we know better. But in recent years, David Bowie, the rock-and-roll singer; Jack Kemp, the Buffalo Bills quarterback and politician; Alan Rickman, the actor; Donna Summer, the singer; and other celebrities have died of cancer. Specifically what kind of cancer has rarely been made public though. Obituary writers at the *New York Times,* the *Washington Post,* and other newspapers routinely ask for the cause of death, but the families of the deceased refuse to name the specific form of cancer at least 15 percent of the time.

Mom took a final look at Cole's portrait and wheeled Eric back toward the elevators. Up on the third floor, at the far end, stood the isolator units. Even on a quiet night at the hospital, they remained off-limits to unscheduled visitors. Adult leukemia patients and those with advanced tumors took up the fourth floor. In silence, Mom and Eric passed a few of those rooms, where the occasional television glowed blue-white or a distant radio could be heard. The few nurses on duty for the holiday only nodded as they passed another station desk. On the night before Christmas, the hospital remained quiet and serene, empty except for a distant conversation and the warm air echoing through the ducts. Up and down the empty hallways they went—their version of stepping out, hitting the town, going as far afield as the facility design and circumstance allowed on this evening. My mother had to know that her son's health remained precarious as best, that such an opportunity might never come along again.

When the impromptu tour was ended, they rode the elevator alone back to the fifth floor and pediatrics.

Eric whispered, "You know what, Mom?"

"What's that, hon?"

"We're about the only ones here."

"Seems to be."

"That means I must be really sick this time."

32

Eric was discharged on January 16, 1973. The chemotherapy drugs appeared to once again have worked their magic. However, six days later, he could barely get out of bed, and Mom drove him back to Roswell Park, where he went straight to what Mom called "The Purple Room"—the place where severely sick kids were quartered.

To reach the Purple Room, one came off the elevators on the fifth floor and turned right, going past the playroom. At the end of the hall, near the nursing station, one took another right, and that's where the room, perhaps only 10 by 12 feet, could be found. It was almost a primitive precursor to the isolation wards used on the lower floors at Roswell Park.

Photos of family and friends were taped to the garish-colored walls. Among them soon were two black-and-white photos of Jim Schoenfeld: one the standard portrait found in the Sabres' media guide and the other of the redheaded defenseman in action.

"The kid idolizes that hockey player," the nurses whispered to each other, and soon plans were afoot. One of the nurses was either dating or knew somebody who was going out with the young star defenseman for the Sabres.

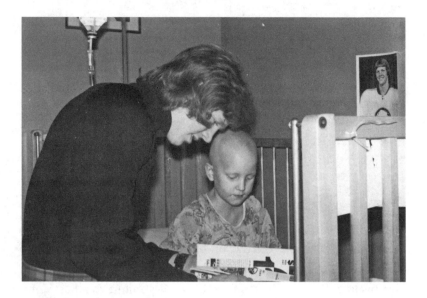

A few days later, dressed in blue turtleneck and plaid pants, Jim Schoenfeld himself paid my brother a visit. As the nurses chatted excitedly, Eric sat upright in a bed with wooden slats front and back and sliding metal gates along the side. IVs were duct-taped to the walls.

This was one of the player's first visits to a local hospital, and Schoenfeld hesitated in the doorway, not sure what to expect. A gaunt kid dressed in a blue hospital gown, with no hair, greeted him. The hockey player blinked and then entered the room with a wide grin.

In photographs taken by my mother, Eric's red lips were about the only color he still exhibited by this point. The rest of him had grown pale to the point of being translucent, and for the first time, his eyes were beginning to lose that knowing sparkle. The visit hadn't been a total surprise. Eric knew something was up when he heard the nurses talking outside his room the day before.

The hockey player brought Eric a transistor radio, the Sabres' yearbook, and a stick signed by the team. He asked my brother what position he played, and Eric replied, "Wing, but I don't score many goals."

"Neither do I," Schoenfeld smiled. Perhaps the star defenseman was being modest. After all, he had scored twice in the weeks leading up to the visit. Still, he would never be mistaken for a scorer and would net no more than nine goals in any season of his fourteen-year NHL career.

Together, Eric and Schoenfeld flipped through the Sabres' yearbook as my mother and several of the nurses watched, almost holding their breath at the moment. Schoenfeld asked to see some of the pictures Eric had drawn. Several were of his family—all of us out on the boat.

"You're a good artist," he said.

"I like to draw," Eric replied. "It helps me think."

Before Schoenfeld left, he switched on the radio, adjusting the dial to the Sabres' flagship station. "That way you can hear how I do," the player said.

"I'll be listening," Eric smiled.

"I'll see if I can score one for you," Schoenfeld added. "I'm not making any guarantees, remember. You and I seem to have the same kind of luck around the net."

The visit lasted maybe a half hour, and when it ended, the radio was placed on a nearby table. The dial was still set to WGR-AM, the Sabres' station.

A few nights later, the Sabres were on the road, playing in Chicago. The host Blackhawks dominated the action, outshooting the Sabres 33–21 for the game, and they took control midway through the third period, scoring two goals within forty-two seconds to take the lead. With less than a minute left in the contest,

Schoenfeld broke the shutout, scoring his fourth and what would be his final goal of the season. Was my brother listening? Nobody knows for sure, but he did have the transistor radio near his bed at Roswell Park.

In the last days of February, Eric's temperature began to spike in increasing intervals. He was treated with more chemotherapy drugs, "without any response," doctors wrote. On March 1, 1973, he became disoriented, and he died of hemorrhage and blood poisoning at 11:25 p.m. the next evening. At the time of his death, Eric was ten years old and weighed 72 pounds. Further examinations found that leukemia had infiltrated several organs and his bone marrow.

The radio and the hockey stick signed by the Sabres team came home to Canal Road with my parents on March 3, 1973. That was a Saturday, and the day began with fog and rain. But by mid-morning, the sun had broken through, with the wind growing out of the southeast and temperatures rising well into the fifties. Susan realized that Eric had died because Mom and Dad were home instead of at the hospital. She went around, awakening the rest of us. With the sun rising into the early March sky, melting the last of the winter snow, she led the little kids on a walk.

"We took off our shoes," she later told me, "and waded in the mud puddles on the gravel pit road."

DECADES LATER, I found myself at the Verizon Center in downtown Washington, D.C., waiting for the New York Rangers to finish practice. It was an off-day before they resumed their playoff series against the hometown Capitals. I was writing a preview about the next game, and as the players began to come off the ice, I started to trail them toward the visitors' locker room. Yet as I took one last look back toward the ice, I saw a tall figure in dark sweats who wasn't wearing a helmet. He shot puck after puck at the top corners of the net. His hair had dulled with the passing years, but it still held a hint of that distinctive reddish hue.

I turned and stepped onto the bench, waving in his direction. Jim Schoenfeld gave me a curious look, before skating over. He didn't recognize me, and why would he? We had talked only once after Eric's death, and that was years ago, when he was playing. Still, as soon as I told him my name, he nodded.

"I remember," he said, his gloved hand resting atop his long hockey stick. "Your brother was about the bravest kid I ever met." We stood there for a moment, not sure what else to say.

"The family's good?" Schoenfeld asked. "Your mother? She was such a fine person. Always with a smile on her face."

"She's still going strong. Everyone's doing fine."

Schoenfeld nodded again. At the far end of the ice, the rink doors opened and the Zamboni prepared to resurface the ice. The team practice was over, with another game scheduled for tomorrow night.

"Your brother," Schoenfeld said, "deserved a lot better."

With that he skated away, shooting the remaining pucks into the net as the Zamboni began to make its rounds, laying down a new layer of fresh ice.

33

When I was sixteen, less than a year before my brother died, I announced that I wasn't interested in joining the family engineering firm. I knew I wasn't cut out for that line of work.

In eighth grade, I had struggled mightily in algebra. I never should have been taking the subject that early in school, and one could argue that my mind would never be ready for unknown values and balanced equations. My algebra teacher was also the high school cross-country coach. A few weeks into the school year, he told me to join him after the final bell. I thought it would be a study session, one of many that I needed. Even though we did go over a few exercises, the conversation soon turned to my immediate future.

"I'll make sure you pass this class," he told me. "I'll do what I can to give you a decent shot at the New York State Regents exam."

That sounded great to me.

"But you'll need to hold up your end of the deal," he added.

I had no idea what he was talking about.

"I saw you at the Junior High Track and Field Day. You're pretty fast. What would you think about running for me?"

I agreed, and I would run on the Roy-Hart team and even become captain of the track squad as a senior. In return, the coach made sure I somehow passed algebra.

When I left the classroom that afternoon, hurrying to make the late bus home, I remember thinking, "This is how the world works. You make the best deal you can."

When I told my family that I wasn't cut out to be a civil engineer, the dinner table briefly grew quiet. Grandpa Lee was especially disappointed. That said, the world soon moved ahead. After all, there were much bigger issues at stake at the time.

Would I have reconsidered, even become an engineer, if my brother had lived? All I know is that Jim Harrison, the novelist, once said that a family accident or tragedy can force a person to move ahead "without compromise."

Ironically, Grandpa Lee, the one who had founded the family engineering firm in 1940 and built it into a company with more than two hundred employees today, soon became one of my biggest backers. When I got my first media pass to cover a Buffalo Sabres game for *Hockey* magazine, he insisted I show him the piece of cardboard with the team insignia and its string of twine to attach it to a shirt buttonhole or belt loop. What I was trying to do, to become a sportswriter, had gained a measure of legitimacy in his eyes.

34

Decades later, when my wife and I neared the end of our fellowship year in Ann Arbor, my son, Chris, was doing much better. Whether it was the doses of Albuterol or the warmer weather,
he became a whirlwind of activity, riding his big-wheel tricycle on
the gymnasium floor at the downtown YMCA, where he attended
preschool, and he kept up with the big kids through the concrete
courtyards of married student housing at Michigan.

One day I took him to the noontime public skate at Yost Ice
Arena. My parents, when they were students in Ann Arbor, had
gone to other events in that brick barn of a building. Nearly a half
century later, I purchased a partial season ticket plan for the men's
hockey team, and we cheered them on to the national championship that year. Several times we went to the Wolverines' practice at
Yost, and Coach Red Berenson took a shine to Chris, making sure
such top players as Brendan Morrison, the star forward, and Marty
Turco, the goalie, stopped by to talk with him.

Chris could barely skate back then. If anything, he reminded me
of myself when I first took up the game when the Kenan Arena
opened in Lockport back in 1968. I laced the pint-sized hockey
skates onto Chris's feet (never figure skates in our family), and
we made our way with halting steps toward the glimmering ice

surface with the gigantic blue block M in the middle of it. My plan was to begin slow, perhaps make it as far as the team benches a quarter of the way around and take a break. The plan was to coach Chris through the skating motion—push and glide—to point out how different it is compared to walking and certainly running.

We both wore winter jackets, and Chris had on snow pants and a helmet. We stepped onto the ice, merging into the slow conga line of skaters moving counterclockwise around the ice surface. We would just fit in, take our time, I told myself. Yet soon Chris broke away from me, digging hard between the flowing ranks of the other skaters, somehow staying on his feet with choppy strides, moving toward center ice. Sometimes figure skaters practiced their jumps and turns in this quieter area. On this afternoon, thankfully, it was open ice once we had passed the skate guards.

Soon I caught up to Chris, gliding alongside him in case he fell. "Where you going in such a hurry, Tiger?" I asked.

He didn't answer as he dug in his blades, making for the very center of the ice surface. A few feet from the block M, Chris dove headfirst, like a base runner determined to steal second, and then rolled onto his back as he came to rest in the middle of the giant letter at center ice. He gazed up at the rafters, where the banners of Michigan's championship seasons hung, and began to laugh.

"What are you doing?" I asked, kneeling down beside him.

"From the first game we ever saw here," my four-year-old explained, "I've wanted to do that. Now I have." Both of us laughed, and I knew exactly how he felt and why he had done it.

For there is something about a fresh sheet of ice, gleaming in the light as it hardens after a new coat of Zamboni water. It beckons you, drawing you from the safer quarters on the other side of the boards. It can beguile and hypnotize you into taking the first shaky steps onto its clear surface. It smiles again as you take hold of the boards and then push free, seeing where the skate blades can take you. With every halting stride, the frozen glittering mirror urges you to cross over from what you are familiar with to what you might know, what you might even become.

35

"I spoke with Dr. Pinkel a few weeks ago," I told Lucius Sinks.

"That right?" the doctor said. "Where's he at now?"

"Cal Poly, where he teaches biological sciences. He told me that he tries to swim every day. And he's got sixteen grandchildren now."

Sinks smiled. "Good for him."

"He was asking me how old I was when my brother died."

"That right?"

"Yeah, as I've told you, I was ten years old when he was diagnosed and seventeen, a junior in high school, when Eric died. Pinkel said that's something you never forget. How it can change your life forever."

Sinks nodded, "It does, doesn't it?"

After our lunch, on the drive home from Charlottesville, I remembered a December night in 1977. Earlier that day, we had buried my Grandma Bunny in a small cemetery outside of Lockport. Despite being a chronic smoker, she had lived until the age of seventy-eight. Her funeral and Eric's couldn't have been more different. Grandma Bunny's had the traditional organ music and hymns, and the line of cars heading to the cemetery. At Eric's, each of us brought something special of his—teddy bears, drawing books, the jacket he wore sailing. I remember carrying one of his hockey skates. Still, to me, a funeral was a funeral.

The evening after we buried my grandmother, a steady drizzle was falling by the time I turned off the New York State Thruway and sped up the hill to the Syracuse University campus. It was Saturday night, the last one before final exams began the next week, and there were plenty of people out as I parked on East Adams Street. Pulling my trench coat tight, I made my way to the student lounge. Syracuse University didn't have a student union back then, but I wanted to be around people, hear them talk and carry on, even though I wasn't ready to say much myself.

My grandmother's passing came less than four years after my brother's. In between those seismic events, my best friend from high school, John Douglas, had died in a car crash on Route 31, east of Middleport. That occurred two months after Eric's death.

The phone call that night came after dinner, as I was watching a hockey game from Toronto, waiting for the inevitable. Somehow I went to school the next day. There were no grief counselors back then, and I later won the school citizenship award, which had been started in John's honor. Through it all, I felt as if I was stumbling through life, worried about holding on to what was left of me.

Inside the student lounge, I found a small table in the back. I had come on the off chance that a woman I was seeing might be here too. Jacqui Salmon regularly worked at the student lounge. We had met at the *Daily Orange*, the student newspaper, and I loved it when I could make her laugh. Then I remembered that she had a formal at Alpha Phi tonight, her sorority next door. Once we had talked about my attending as her date—before I had to head home for another family funeral.

I sat at the empty table, thinking about the people I had lost in recent years—my brother, my friend John, and now my grandmother.

While I knew other people had it much worse, I couldn't determine how anyone kept going through situations like this. How they found it in themselves to dream and smile when they had to feel so overwhelmed and so alone.

The crowd at the bar grew to three- to four-people deep as the clock on the wall swept past eleven at night. The laughter and commotion drifted back to me as I stood up and began to pull my coat on. That's when Jacqui came through door.

She was wearing a long black gown with a bodice of roses and platform heels. Her hair was pulled back into a tight bun, with a few wisps swept free by the wind and drizzle. As I waved, taking a step or two toward her, how I wanted to slide those stray strands back into place.

"I was hoping you'd be here," she told me in a breathless voice. "I skipped out on him."

"Who?"

"My date, of course. Oh, God, he'll never forgive me. But who cares? I told him I had to study for exams and went out the back door."

I began to laugh.

"You look terrible," she said. "Your face is so pale." She turned to the bartender, a big blond guy named Jeff. "Get Wendel a drink," she snapped. The two of them worked together, so he ignored the multitude of orders to deliver us two cognacs.

We returned to my empty table in the back, holding hands.

"Talk to me," Jacqui said. "Just tell me what's on your mind. You know I'll listen. Just talk—tell me anything at all."

So I told her how much I missed my grandmother, how the day had reminded me too much of my brother and my best friend, and how Lockport, down to Olcott, and the waters of Lake Ontario seemed so haunted now. How we used to sail all the way to

Toronto, daring to make another crossing from one side of that wide expanse of water to the other. How we used to play hockey at the local rink or on the pond behind our house. How I so loved playing softball on the West Bluff, a short bike ride from the harbor, and how we had once tuned in the radio stations from Toronto and Buffalo, and how, if the conditions were right, we could dial in Detroit, Chicago, and St. Louis too. How all of it had been enough for years and years and years. It had been enough—until now.

"Why is it that everybody I love dies?" I asked her.

In reply, Jacqui brought my hand to her face and ran it gently along her cheek.

"It's OK," she said. "Believe me, it's going to be OK."

36

"Soon after your brother," Sinks said when we met again, "so much of what we've been talking about at Roswell Park began to change."

Indeed, the Hollands, James and Jimmie, would soon leave for a year in the Soviet Union. President Richard Nixon took great pride in his foreign policy, sometimes to the detriment of his domestic programs. In 1972, not long after signing the National Cancer Act, he again turned his attention overseas, this time to the Cold War.

As Holland remembered it, the president "and Leonid Brezhnev tried to put aside the notion of dropping atomic bombs on each other and agreed that finding a cure for cancer would be mutually beneficial. . . . I think that perhaps the best diplomacy that the United States can offer is through its health services. Because every country really wants its people to be healthy, every sensible citizen deplores the fact that people die from preventable causes, and so I think doctors turn out to be very good diplomats."

And Holland was about to get his chance at being a medical diplomat. Nixon and Brezhnev decided that the two countries would exchange doctors for eight months—a goodwill gesture that might result in medical progress.

C. Gordon Zubrod at the National Cancer Institute was put in charge of finding an American doctor to go to the Soviet Union. Holland was enlisted to help select a candidate, but nobody in the ALGB was really interested.

Those at Roswell Park were more concerned with what was happening in their own backyard at the time. The money that had flowed for decades from the state capital in Albany had begun to slow. Governor Nelson Rockefeller, who had done his part to build Roswell Park into a topflight research hospital, soon stepped down and eventually become vice president under the new president, Gerald Ford.

Zubrod continued to call Holland. "Have you found somebody to send yet to Russia?" After several calls, and due in large part to the changes on the horizon in Buffalo, Holland asked his wife, "How about us?"

Jimmie Holland agreed, so the Hollands and their children left Buffalo for a year in the Soviet Union. While they were there, James Holland taught the doctors in that country about advances in chemotherapy, using equipment so antiquated that he felt that he was back in his medical school days. Jimmie Holland worked with the Russians about how they defined schizophrenia, a diagnosis sometimes used to imprison dissidents there. Their children shared two bedrooms, the girls in one room, the boys in the other.

While his family was overseas, James Holland received the Albert Lasker Basic Medical Research Award for his work in the treatment of acute leukemia in children. The Hollands missed the ceremony, but the time away gave them the chance to plan their next career move. Upon their return to this country, they resettled in New York City, with James at Mount Sinai and Jimmie at Sloan Kettering. Neither of them would work in Buffalo again.

Sinks would soon follow them to the East Coast. After Nixon's resignation in 1974, there was a heightened desire for transparency at all levels of government in light of the Watergate scandal. This newfound fervor spun out in unexpected directions, sometimes with dire consequences. Hugh Carey, who succeeded Rockefeller as the governor of New York, signed a directive in May 1976 that ordered state employees earning more than $30,000 a year to detail their personal finances, including outside income. Originally designed for policy-making public officials, it was soon applied to the scientists and researchers at Roswell Park, which received public funds.

Fifteen department heads at Roswell called the new policy an invasion of privacy and eventually filed suit against executive order no. 10. None of the doctors was more vocal than Sinks for what he then termed "the callous attitude of the state towards cancer researchers."

Only months before, Sinks and his colleagues had published a new study in which forty out of forty-two children with leukemia were shown to be in remission three years after the new treatments were deployed. Even though Sinks and several of his colleagues made more than $30,000 a year, they claimed they were not in policy-making positions and had no conflict of interest.

The *Courier-Express*, the morning newspaper in Buffalo, disagreed, and in a lead editorial, under the headline "State Doctors Should Bare Finances," it said that the doctors "should be held accountable."

The *Buffalo Evening News* called the situation a "morale problem for Roswell" and said the measure would damage the hospital's "ability to recruit top-flight researchers in today's increasingly stiff competition with a growing number of other leading private and university research agencies."

Dr. Gerald Murphy, the new director at Roswell Park, sided with the governor and New York State. "I don't have any problems publishing my assets," he told *Science* magazine. "The public is asking for reassurance that nothing is going on that's wrong in state institutions. We're going to see more of this kind of thing, not less."

His comments angered many of the hospital's top doctors, and they filed a lawsuit in Erie County court. There, Executive Order No. 10 would later be deemed unconstitutional. "The plaintiffs are employed at Roswell Park Memorial Institute in a noncompetitive class dealing with cancer research and surgery, cancer medical treatment, biophysics, biology, and research science," the verdict read. "They are not an administrative, confidential, managerial policy making class where a potential conflict of interest might be involved. They are valuable research scientists."

By then Sinks had left Buffalo, taking a new position at the Georgetown University School of Medicine in Washington, D.C. "We always felt that we had a good chance at winning in court," he said. "But when your own director comes out publicly against you, what can you do? I just decided it was best to move on—to leave Roswell Park."

I told Sinks that I couldn't believe how quickly it ended. "That meant that the hospital lost the heads of its adult and pediatric wings, you and Holland, within a few months," I said.

"True, and many others left, too. Sometimes that's the way it goes."

Around us another lunch hour at the Boar's Head Inn had come and gone. Together we rose and walked across the restaurant to retrieve our coats from the small closet near the hostess station.

Vincristine
Prednisone
Methotrexate
6-MP

Total Therapy
Daunomycin
Cytoxan
Lomustine
Radiation
Methotrexate injections in intermediate dosages

One could almost repeat the procedures, some kind of strange medical mantra, with each step we took.

For nearly eight years, this swirl of meds used by those at Roswell Park was enough to keep my brother alive. Even though many of the medical personnel no longer called western New York home, the ALGB clinical trials went on. The leukemia doctors stayed in touch, regularly debating about the latest procedures and meds. After so many years together, perhaps they knew no other way.

Study No. 7611, which began a few years after my brother died, continued as "a straightforward comparison" between varying doses of methotrexate given via spinal injections and cranial irradiation. By the mid-1970s, it was generally accepted that radiation should be used only when there was no other alternative to curbing cancer in the central nervous system. Although higher doses of methotrexate did substantially lessen the cancer found in the brain and other areas of the body, once again doctors were reminded that to kill 99.9 percent of the cancer wasn't enough. If any leukemia cells remained, the cancer could return.

The riddle continued about how best to move more medicine past the blood–brain barrier or interface. Decades before, blue dye injected into the bloodstream of a laboratory animal was found to have eventually spread to other tissues of the body except the brain and spinal cord. That's when scientists fully recognized the blood–brain barrier and how it allows some materials to cross and denies others access. Its function is to protect the brain and surrounding area from foreign substances in the blood—even the drugs that target cancer.

In Study No. 7611, the leukemia doctors began to deploy intermediate doses of methotrexate. The key was to administer no more than 500 milligrams per square meter of body surface. In this case, a large, quick dosage amount wasn't necessarily the answer. Perhaps less could be more, allowing enough medicine to move past the blood–brain barrier.

The new approach of intermediate doses soon showed promise. Several hundred children and adolescents participated in a study, and their progress was followed for the next twenty years. Not only did the patients receiving intermediate dosages of methotrexate see no major drop in IQ, they also had no reported instances of secondary cancers. The leukemia could be kept at bay without the often crippling effects of radiation. In the last line of the article that appeared in March 1983, Freeman wrote that intermediate dosages of methotrexate—used intravenously over a longer period of time, complemented with spinal injections—"may replace the need for cranial irradiation in many children with ALL."

In a 1997 follow-up study, coauthored by Freeman, James Holland, Lucius Sinks, and others, the evidence was overwhelmingly positive. The survivors of clinical trial No. 7611, 110 patients in total, were now studied as young adults, something that would have bordered on the impossible a generation before. By then it had been conclusively determined that cranial radiation did "adversely affect intelligence" and that intermediate doses of methotrexate were a much better way to control relapses.

With more young patients moving into remission, the focus shifted to ensuring that they were able to enjoy life to its fullest. Gregory Armstrong at St. Jude said that the use of cranial radiotherapy in ALL patients had dropped from 80 percent in the 1970s to less than 20 percent three decades later. Michael Link at Stanford University said that such changes reflected a new focus on the "cost of the cure," in essence, what patients have to endure to stay alive.

"Given the increasing cure rate," Freeman wrote in the landmark 1983 study, "the quality of life in survivors of ALL has become an important issue."

Professions have different ways of getting the word out, forming a paper trail of record. Not that long ago, it was in letters and even journals. Today, of course, it is in email and even on Twitter. For doctors, what carries the most weight is the list of references, scientific papers, and articles that appear in such publications as *The Lancet, Health Affairs,* and the *New England Journal of Medicine.* Here is where the victories and next steps, the triumphs and breakthroughs, are duly recorded. That can leave a novice often lost and even overwhelmed, sifting through the terminology and procedures to find the golden nuggets of information and promise.

So it was with the paper entitled "Intermediate-Dose Methotrexate versus Cranial Irradiation in Childhood Acute Lymphoblastic Leukemia: A Ten-Year Follow-Up," tracking patients in Study No. 7611. In the conclusion, one line stood out for me: "By the year 2010, one in 250 adults between the ages of 20 and 45 in the United States will be a survivor of childhood cancer."

There it was, with no hyperbole or bluster. A simple line that indicated how far the medical world has come, how much we have learned, since my brother was first diagnosed with acute lymphoblastic leukemia. Now one in 250 will be a cancer survivor.

The leukemia doctors are uneasy talking about breakthroughs. They really don't view the world in such terms and were more focused on the day to day and what could be done with the clinical trial or the next drug at their disposal. In doing so, they made key advances in cancer medicine. After realizing that there were no magic bullets, that one drug couldn't cure this form of cancer by itself, they used chemotherapy drugs in combination, deploying them to target DNA replication, eliminating cancer cells "roughly in proportion to how fast they are replicating."

The story of the blood centrifuge machine, the IBM 2990 and 2991, underscored their work ethic and ability to regularly think outside the box. Many of us daydream about devices or methods that can make our jobs easier. Few of us sit down the next day and begin working on making such things a reality.

Then there was the use of methotrexate to keep patients in remission. Until that point, higher dosages and the increased use of chemotherapy drugs had been proven, time and again, to be the most successful approaches. That the doctors could go in a different direction, with so much at stake, after young patients had been moved into remission shows, I believe, real courage and genius. This trio of advances changed the medical world forever.

37

By our last summer together on the boat, I could pretty much predict when my father would sing out, "Man overboard." It was a ruse by then, a simple drill to keep us on our toes about the dangers of sailing across miles of open water, well offshore.

To this day, Eric is the only member of our family to be in the "Wet Pants Club," his name on the pegboard at Olcott Yacht Club after he walked off the end of the dock when nobody was looking. He was five years old or so back then—when he and my youngest brother, Bryan, always wore life jackets within sight of the water.

On this late August afternoon, we angled away from the American shore, hardening up into the wind. The bluffs above Olcott harbor rose behind us, and I somehow knew Dad couldn't resist. Sitting in the shade of the foredeck with my sister, Susan, I saw him steal a step toward the lazarette near the engine controls. He reached down and grasped one of the life jackets stored there and flung it over his shoulder. With a splash, the orange flotation device landed far behind us, in our wake.

"Man overboard," he shouted and stepped away from the wheel, eager to see how quickly we would react.

"For God's sake," Susan muttered as we bounded down into the cockpit, past my mother and the younger kids, all heads and chatter now. My middle brother, Chris, had already slackened the mainsail, and Susan moved to do the same with the jib sheet.

"Ready about," I shouted as I took the helm.

"Ready," sang out the others, even though they didn't have much to do, except keep an eye on the orange life jacket bobbing well behind us.

"Hard-a-lee," I ordered and steered the vessel up into the wind. Soon we came around and headed in the opposite direction, bearing down on the life jacket.

"Watch your speed," Dad said as we approached the floating orange object.

Always a step ahead, Susan had the boat hook out, extended to its full length, ready to snare our prize.

"You don't want to run him over," Dad warned. "Never a good idea on a rescue mission."

Without needing to be told, my siblings slackened the sails, letting them flap in the wind, as I pulled alongside. I kept the bobbing target to windward, and Susan reached over to snare the life jacket, with Chris alongside to help. The little guys, Eric and Bryan, always wanted a better look, and they scrambled out from the shadow of the cabin and hung beside me. Once we had retrieved the jacket, Eric and Bryan often had their hands on the helm—either a wooden tiller stick or later on a gleaming stainless steel wheel. And I would let go, allowing them to steer awhile.

Dad invariably mentioned how long it took us—he always glanced at his watch during our impromptu rescue missions. Our best effort was maybe three minutes, which I thought was pretty good. Still, Dad would point out that in the chill of early spring or late autumn, a person could soon die of hypothermia in these waters. The goal of "Man Overboard" was to be faster, always faster. You never knew when lives could be at stake.

A FEW YEARS AGO, Mom brought out several of Eric's things that she had kept stored away. They included his black, fake alligator wallet held together with a snap button clasp. Several of us, my parents and brother Chris, gathered around as we sorted through its few contents. There was his cut-out identification card for *Scholastic* magazine, filled out in large block-printed letters. Two pennies were in the coin purse, one dated 1964, the other 1970. In the side flap, a sticker announced that he was a junior fire marshal at school. The other side flap held three photographs, the small class shots that are taken every year, usually in the fall.

One was of Eric, his face swollen by the latest round of chemotherapy treatments. Even though he had put on weight, he looked dapper in a blue mock turtleneck. The others were of Paul Glazer, his best friend at the time, and a beautiful little girl with blonde hair wearing a freshly ironed plaid dress. Eric had been smitten with her, and now none of us could remember her name.

Mom had also kept several of Eric's report cards. Throughout it all, he put up good grades—often Es for Excellent progress in art, music, and physical education, and in the 90s for language arts, social studies, arithmetic, and science. Those were the headings back then, before many of the same disciplines earned such designations as interpersonal skills, interpretive history, and accelerated math.

Everyone knows someone who made it through school missing only a few days due to colds or other illness. In high school, I had a friend who didn't miss a single day from seventh through twelfth grade. He was as regular as the sun in the morning. If school opened its doors, he was there, and it wasn't because he necessarily enjoyed the classroom that much. It had become a point of honor with him, a streak to maintain no matter how much he may have felt like staying home and hiding under the covers some days.

Of course, Eric never had any chance at an unblemished slate when it came to attendance. In the 1969–1970 school year alone, as a student in Mrs. Thompson's first grade class, he missed more than twenty-four days of school due to the trips to Roswell Park. By the first half of the 1972–1973 school year, when things went downhill, he missed eighteen half-days in the first quarter and a stunning sixty-five in the second quarter. Despite the time away from school, his grades ranged from 90 to 95 in all subjects, and his only S for Satisfactory came in PE. In nearly everything else, he was given E for Excellent.

"Eric is a very good student," Mrs. Brown wrote in the teacher's comments for the first period. "He is a joy in the classroom." My mother had signed on the line requiring a parent's signature.

At the end of the second period, Mrs. Brown added, "I have evaluated Eric with the marks that I have this time. We miss Eric's joy in our classroom. We hope he comes back soon." The report card went unsigned this time around, and he never returned to Gasport Elementary, the low-slung building along Route 31.

A few months after Eric's death, my parents received a letter from Principal Gibbs. He told them that a print of a painting entitled "Homeward Bound" had been installed to remember Eric in the corridor of Wing A near the fourth grades. It hung there for several years before being replaced by newer works.

38

Sometimes I wonder what kind of person my brother would have grown up to be if he had lived. My siblings have their own ideas and projections.

My brother Bryan remembered that Eric "was wicked smart and could have been anything he wanted to be. I always thought he would have probably been an MD-PhD and done research in medicine or engineering. He loved learning, and I was always amazed at how well he did in school considering how much school he had to miss at certain times for treatments. He was like a sponge and could grasp bigger, more intricate concepts with relative ease."

The hockey stick signed by the Buffalo Sabres today hangs on Bryan's office wall.

Chris said he thinks about Eric almost every day and believes that his "legacy provided a sense of reality for all of us: Don't take anything for granted. No petty arguments. Try to be kind and considerate to one another, just like he was." He pointed out that Paul Glazer, Eric's best friend, has his own hedge fund on Wall Street. "Both were similar in mental horsepower and demeanor," Chris said, "and it's hard to believe that Eric would not have done great things."

My youngest sister, Amy, was only five years old when Eric died. During my brother's final months, she attended preschool at the Kenan Center and went over to various friends' homes afterward. I picked her up after high school and track practice.

"When asked what kind of person my brother would have grown up to be, I have trouble answering that," Amy said. "At five years old, I was much too young to form that sort of idea. But I do know this, based on what my older siblings and my parents told me: he would have been a caring person."

Susan was closer to Eric than the rest of her siblings. She married a man whose birthday is on November 21, one day after Eric's. Her husband, Richard, and Eric both enjoy solving puzzles, figuring things out, and telling a good story, and both are willing to sacrifice their other needs for the good of others.

If Eric had lived he would have been in high school during the recession of the 1980s when our parents remortgaged the house to keep the family engineering firm afloat, Susan said. Eric, more than the rest of us, would have been enthralled with the first home computer, a Franklin ACE, that Dad brought home in the early 1980s.

"In the latitude to determine my dead brother's life trajectory, I cast him as the missing puzzle piece," Susan told me. "I think he might have chosen the role that the rest of us turned our backs on and become the third generation at Wendel Engineers."

For myself, I believe that Eric wouldn't have had any reluctance at all about returning to the cruel though promising world that tried to save him. When I close my eyes, I can picture him as a doctor or researcher, someone wearing the white medical coat over a shirt and tie.

Over the years, so much can fade away and be forgotten. Looking through the old family photos, some of them nearly a half-century old now, can become one surprise after another. I'd forgotten that Eric parted his reddish-brown hair on the right. How he liked to button his shirts up tight to the collar, looking so professional. How when the rest of us were always ready to mug for the camera, posing as pirates or renegades, he would be in our midst, usually looking directly at the lens, revealing only a wry smile.

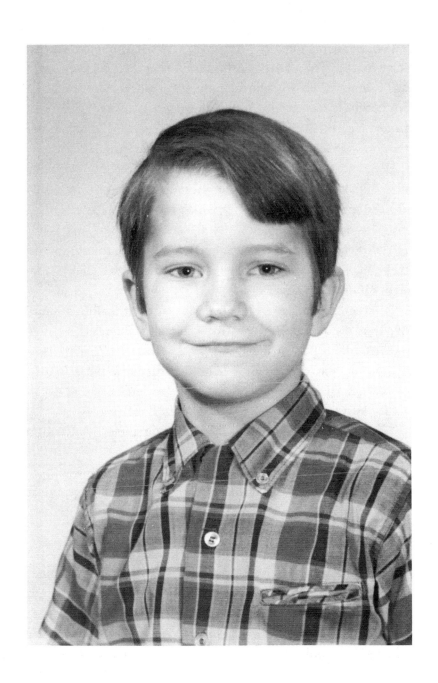

I once took my son, Chris, on a trip back to my hometown, just the two of us. We played a round of golf at the Lockport Town and Country Club, where my Grandpa Lee was remembered by a few of the old-timers. On our last afternoon, I drove to Olcott and parked near the yacht club, and Chris and I walked to the end of the port-side pier, the one with the flashing red light.

None of us Wendel kids owns a sailboat larger than a dinghy now. Still, when we approach the shoreline, each of us invariably glances upward, checking to see which way the breeze is coming from on this day, judging how best to set our sails.

"So when we came out of the harbor, we would round up into the wind," I told Chris. "From here it would be seven to eight hours across, if the wind held."

"To where?" Chris asked, gazing at the far horizon. It was a hazy August afternoon, and none of Toronto's tall buildings was visible on the far side of the lake.

"All the way across," I replied. "Another crossing to the far side of the lake. Usually to Toronto."

"Toronto, Canada?"

"That's right. It's a straight shot across on a good day, with a steady wind."

"And you were on how big a boat?"

"We began aboard the 24-footer, *Ibeecha*, and our biggest boat ever was 30-foot."

"And your whole family went?"

"Yep, eight of us. We all had jobs to do."

Chris considered this as we gazed on Lake Ontario and the miles of open water between us and the horizon. He glanced at Olcott's small harbor and then back to the big lake, where no other vessel, not even a mighty lake freighter, was visible on this summer afternoon. He only nodded, both of us momentarily lost in our thoughts. Then we turned and together walked back down the pier to our car and the ride home.

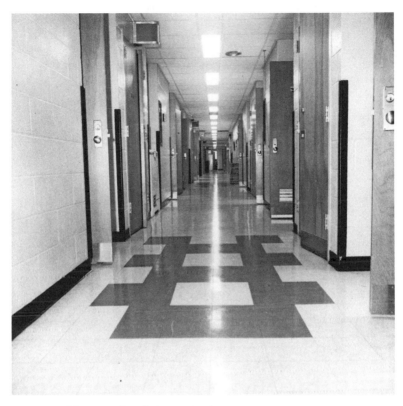

Courtesy of the Roswell Park Cancer Institute.

Acknowledgments

A t first, this book appears to be a departure from my previous works, most of which dealt with sports and history. Yet
as my friend Howard Mansfield points out, "You're always writing
about these kinds of groups and individuals. Those who take on
and try to overcome great odds." So it was with this determined
cadre of doctors— Donald Pinkel, James Holland, Jerry Yates, and
Lucius Sinks. If there was a Mount Rushmore of cancer research,
they would be on it. I am thankful for their guidance and patience.

Driving to Charlottesville, Virginia, to visit with Dr. Sinks became
a welcome regular event in researching this book. He assembled the
flowchart of my brother's meds, lent me textbooks, and directed me
toward the crucial reports that were written during this golden age
of medical discovery. His advice and counsel were invaluable.

Part of the riddle of doing any book is finding the right home for
it. Thankfully, I fell in with Cornell University Press. From the first
time that we talked about the project, on a rainy night after his class
in Alexandria, Virginia, Dean J. Smith understood what this book
could really be. He brought in Frances Benson, Nathan Gemignani,
James Lance, Martyn Beeny, and Suzanne Gordon, who urged me
to underscore the medical advances during this period as well as
my family story. Just as important, Meagan Dermody, Julie Nemer,

Marie Flaherty-Jones, and Sara Ferguson moved everything with style and grace through the production process. Thanks to their efforts and patience, this is a far better book than when I began.

Back in the day, my brother had many folks looking out for him at Roswell Park. Decades later, I was just as fortunate. Sue Banchich soon became a good friend, as interested in this period in the hospital's history as I was. She put me in touch with many key people, including Jerry Yates, Philip McCarthy, and Martin Brecher, who kindly wrote the foreword. On a windy day in February, I found myself at the Edwin A. Mirand Library in Buffalo. Nancy Cunningham and John Crawford made me feel welcome and led me to several key finds there.

Thanks to Gary Brozek, who read an early version and made several important suggestions. Gary edited my first novel, *Castro's Curveball*, and he is someone I've relied on so much over the years. The same goes for Richard Peabody, the editor of *Gargoyle*, where early chapters appeared. I had several conversations about this project with my longtime friend Bob Reichblum, who enthusiastically urged me to go ahead with it. I am just sorry he didn't live to see the finished book.

Tamara Jones, a marvelous writer and family friend, urged me to jot down whatever came into my head about those family sailing trips. Just to write them down and figure out where such passages fit into the overall narrative later. Initially, I had my doubts about this approach, but it came together, especially in finding the moments or pivot points that Eric shared with those who cared for him in Buffalo.

Special thanks to my students at Johns Hopkins University and to my good friends there: David Everett, Elise Levine, Ed Perlman, Melissa Hendricks, Karen Houppert, Mark Farrington, and Cathy Alter. Our conversations helped me to keep moving ahead.

In the kind of coincidences and serendipitous moments one relies on in the midst of a project like this, my longtime friend Budd

Bailey introduced me to Kathleen Darcy, a professional in this area. Kathleen went to great lengths to explain the medicines and dosages at play here. Paul Goldberg from *The Cancer Letter* was there to answer more of my questions. His publication is a must-read for those interested in the dramatic advances in this field.

My parents and my siblings soon realized how important this project was for me and regularly came to my assistance. My mother put up with my questions and repeatedly peeled back the years, determined to underscore the good times, especially the humorous incidents, amid the array of treatments and procedures at Roswell Park. In taking us out on the waters of Lake Ontario, my father taught us the power of unseen forces and that wide expanses to the horizon are nothing to be feared.

My admiration for my parents only grew as I did the book. Studies show that the death of a child can be devastating to any couple. Divorce rates among bereaved parents are as high as eight times the norm. That said, Jane and Peter Wendel have been married for sixty-one years and remain leaders in the Lockport community, as well as spirited grandparents and now great-grandparents. Their crossing has not been easy, with plenty of choppy seas, but they have never complained.

Every family has a historian and my brother Chris will always be ours. When my memory grew hazy, the pivotal dates and moments somehow remained clear to him. So often I was the beneficiary of his recollections. My brother Bryan and sister Amy, who were closer to Eric in age than I was, explained the family dynamics from that end of the spectrum.

My sister Susan has always been my partner in mischief. When we were just kids, I convinced her to offer up her spare change, and we buried it in a miniature cedar chest in the backyard on Canal Road. Although the companion map was soon lost, I was heartened that somewhere down the hill from the house, near the sandbox, our treasure might someday be found.

In writing the book, I was reminded about the importance of place. In my case, the Kenan Center in Lockport, the north woods of Michigan, the West Bluff along Lake Ontario. In Olcott, we played softball on a parcel of land adjacent to an orchard. A nod of gratitude to the families there and my friends from those times: Bryan Wollenberg, Dan Stein, Kim Miller, Sharon Hewner, Warren Haseley, and Paul Buerger.

In an effort to focus on the present and what is in front of me, I practice with Thu Nguyen at the Mindfulness Practice Center in Oakton, Virginia. While my mind still races along, our conversations about family and our shared world often give me solace.

Michael Shorofsky and his parents, Sheryl and Steve, took time to explain the medical culture to me and how it has changed over the decades. Greg Williamson at Johns Hopkins University told me to read L. E. Sissman, whose poetry influenced me as I was finishing the manuscript. "To see the moon so silver going west." That line will forever remind me of my brother.

Throughout this project, as well as three previous books, my agent Chris Park and the folks at Foundry+Media have been in my corner. I could not have done it without them.

In addition, my good friend Paul Dickson remains a great sounding board for any kind of project. How I love to talk about stories and the world with him.

Finally, thanks to my children, Sarah and Christopher, and my wife, Jacqueline. This project began with a question that I could not fully answer. Now I can only hope that my kids continue to excel in their fields and prove to be as resilient, as determined, and as compassionate as my brother and those who tried to cure him.

Notes

Chapter 1

1 **"Ibeecha!"** Susan Wendel Och, author's interview, August 12, 2014; Chris Wendel, author's interview, September 9, 2013.

3 **". . . the best thing I've ever done."** "Dulles International Airport Terminal Building," *Architect*, March 18, 2015, http://www.architectmagazine.com/project-gallery/dulles-international-airport-terminal-building.

4 **". . . hit me pretty hard"** Peter Wendel, author's interview, May 3, 2013.

5 **"There is no cure for leukemia . . ."** Hazel Fath, *A Dream Come True: The Story of St. Jude Children's Hospital and ALSAC* (Dallas: Taylor Publishing, 1983), 79.

Chapter 2

7 **"Dad, you had a brother . . ."** Sarah Wendel, conversation with the author, October 19, 2013.

8 **After Sarah left that evening . . .** Arnold I. Freeman, Vivian Weinberg, Martin L. Brecher, Barbara Jones, Arvin S. Glicksman, Lucius F. Sinks, Marise Weil, Hansjuerg Pleuss, Juliet Hananian, E. Omer Burgert, Jr., Gerald S. Gilchrist, Thomas Necheles, Michael Harris, Faith Kung, Richard B. Patterson, Harold Maurer, Brigid Leventhal, Louise Chevalier, Edwin Forman, and James F. Holland, "Comparison of Intermediate-Dose Methotrexate with Cranial Irradiation for Post-Induction Treatment of Acute Lymphocytic Leukemia in Children," *New England Journal of Medicine* 308 (1983), http://dx.doi.org/10.1056/NEJM198303033080902.

8 **Pinkel had founded the Department of Pediatrics . . .** For a timeline of the history of Cancer and Leukemia Group B (CALGB), see https://www.calgb.org/Public/about/history.php.

8 **Today, that statistic . . .** Stephen P. Hunger and Charles G. Mullighan, "Acute Lymphoblastic Leukemia in Children," *New England Journal of Medicine* 373 (2015): 1541–52.

9 **If anything, I'm willing . . .** Jack Kerouac, *On the Road* (New York: Signet, 1955), 9.

10 **"Some determined people . . ."** Jerome Yates, author's interview, November 7, 2013.

11 **"You have to remember something . . ."** James Holland, author's interview, November 8, 2013.

Chapter 3

13 **Vincristine comes from the periwinkle plant . . .** Chemocare, "Vincristine," 2017, http://chemocare.com/chemotherapy/drug-info/Vincristine.aspx.

13 **In comparison, prednisone is . . .** Drugs.com, "Prednisone," 2017, https://www.drugs.com/prednisone.html.

14 **Vincristine and prednisone . . .** Kathleen Darcy, author's interview, October 8, 2015; Alfred G. Gilman, Louis S. Goodman, Theodore W. Rall, and Ferid Murad, *The Pharmacological Basis of Therapeutics* (New York: Macmillan, 1985), 1279–82.

14 **Patients in Study No. 6601 . . .** James Holland, author's interview, November 19, 2014; Lucius Sinks, author's interview, February 20, 2015; Jerome Yates, author's interview, August 12, 2014; Vincent T. DeVita, Jr., and Elizabeth DeVita-Raeburn, *The Death of Cancer: After Fifty Years on the Front Lines of Medicine, a Pioneering Oncologist Reveals Why the War on Cancer Is Winnable—and How We Can Get There* (New York: Farrar, Straus and Giroux, 2015), 60–64.

15 **Zubrod, like many of the leukemia doctors . . .** John Laszlo, *The Cure of Childhood Leukemia: Into the Age of Miracles* (New Brunswick, NJ: Rutgers University Press, 1996), 93–107.

16 **"Gordon was the grease . . ."** James Holland, author's interview, November 19, 2014.

16 **"Of course, this was well before . . ."** Donald Pinkel, author's interview, October 13, 2013.

17 **After a study Holland dearly wanted . . .** James Holland, author's interview, November 19, 2014.

17 **"To really do the job . . ."** Donald Pinkel, author's interview, July 22, 2014.

18 **Holland told me that . . .** James Holland, author's interview, November 19, 2014.

18 **"What I see is a patient . . ."** Kathleen Darcy, author's interview, August 16, 2016.

18 **Dad's plan was to sail . . .** Chris Wendel, author's interview, November 14, 2014.

Chapter 4

21 **Pinkel's own health** . . . Mary Pinkel, author's interview, February 3, 2015.

21 **Any notion that his move back** . . . Unless otherwise noted, stories and quotations in this chapter come from the interviews I conducted with Donald Pinkel on October 22, 2013, and July 22, 2014, and from a now-defunct web story, Roswell Park Cancer Institute, "A Sense of Urgency: Donald Pinkel and the Quest to Cure ALL," accessed February 1, 2016, http://www.roswellpark.org/donaldpinkel.

27 **While Pinkel, Holland, and others** . . . Hampton Sides, "Childhood Leukemia Was Practically Untreatable until Dr. Don Pinkel and St. Jude Hospital Found a Cure," *Smithsonian Magazine*, July 2016, http://www.smithsonianmag.com/innovation/childhood-leukemia-untreatable-dr-don-pinkel-st-jude-180959501/.

28 **Pinkel's daughter, Becky, remembered** . . . Becky Pinkel, author's interview, February 4, 2015.

29 **"My dad's patients nearly always died . . ."** Ibid.

Chapter 5

32 **It came with two sails** . . . SailboatData.com, "Shark 24," accessed July 20, 2017, http://sailboatdata.com/viewrecord.asp?class_id=44.

34 **I met Oates once** . . . Joyce Carol Oates, conversation with the author, September 30, 2004.

34 **She had written that the region** . . . Joyce Carol Oates, "American Gothic," *New Yorker*, May 8, 1995, 35, http://www.newyorker.com/magazine/1995/05/08/american-gothic-2.

35 **Eudora Welty once wrote** . . . Eudora Welty, "Place in Fiction," *Collected Essays* (New York, 1994), edited scan, University of Virginia, accessed on November 13, 1995, xroads.virginia.edu/~drbr/welty.txt.

Chapter 6

39 **Warning labels for 6-MP** . . . Chemocare, "6-MP," accessed July 19, 2017, http://chemocare.com/chemotherapy/drug-info/6-mp.aspx.

39 **Cancer cells, especially if they are** . . . Kathleen Darcy, author's interview, October 8, 2015.

40 **"To many in the medical establishment . . ."** Jerome Yates, author's interview, August 12, 2014.

40 **"The sweet meringue . . ."** Jane Wendel, author's interview, March 11, 2015.

42 **After all, the Tibetans asked . . .** Wade Davis, *Into the Silence: The Great War, Mallory, and the Conquest of Everest* (New York: Vintage, 2012), 33.

43 **"That was your family's . . ."** Donald Pinkel, author's interview, July 22, 2014.

Chapter 8

48 **Pinkel knew about the national tragedy . . .** Edwin A. Mirand, *Legacy and History of Roswell Park Cancer Institute, 1898–1998* (Virginia Beach: Donning, 1998), 9–16.

49 **On September 6, 1901 . . .** Sarah Vowell, *Assassination Vacation* (New York: Simon & Schuster, 2006), 193–96.

Chapter 9

52 **"So you made it down from D.C.?"** Lucius Sinks, author's interview, December 6, 2013. All quotations in this chapter are from this interview and the follow-up email.

Chapter 10

58 **Holland told the audience . . .** "New Drug Method Eases Leukemia," *New York Times*, April 10, 1965.

58 **During his presentation . . .** Ibid.

59 **"[It] goes back to an editorial . . ."** James Holland, author's interview, November 19, 2014.

59 **"I have been criticized . . ."** Ibid.

59 **One of the first documented cases . . .** Stories about the origins of leukemia and early attempts at treatments can be found in Eugene W. Straus and Alex Straus, *Medical Marvels: The 100 Greatest Advances in Medicine* (Amherst, NY: Prometheus Books, 2006), 269–70; Malcolm Gladwell, *David and Goliath: Underdogs, Misfits and the Art of Battling Giants* (New York: Little, Brown, 2013), 153–59; John Laszlo, *The Cure of Childhood Leukemia: Into the Age of Miracles* (New Brunswick, NJ: Rutgers University Press, 1996), 7–9.

60 **Today, the American Cancer Society . . .** National Cancer Institute, "What Is Cancer?" 2015, http://www.cancer.gov/about-cancer/what-is-cancer.

60 **Leukemia is the most common . . .** American Association for Cancer Research Foundation, "Cancer Types," n.d., https://www.aacrfoundation.org/CancerTypes/Pages/default.aspx.

61 **That different chemotherapy drugs . . .** NIH Clinical Center, "Dr. James F. Holland Shares Memories of CC's Early Days," accessed July 21, 2017, http://www.cc.nih.gov/about/news/annivers60/holland.shtml.

61 **"That's what we were up against, . . ."** Jerome Yates, author's interview, November 7, 2013.

61 **Leukemia could be beaten . . .** James Holland, author's interview, November 19, 2013.

62 **In the medical journal *Blood*, . . .** William Dameshek, Thomas F. Necheles, Harvey E. Finkel, and Donald M. Allen, "Therapy of Acute Leukemia, 1965," *Blood* 26, no. 2 (1965): 220–25.

62 **Growing up in Buffalo . . .** Saul Wisnia, "Sidney Farber, Chemo Crusader," New York Public Radio Archives and Preservation, March 27, 2015, http://www.wnyc.org/story/sidney-farber-chemo-crusader/.

62 **"I will not injure two children to save one."** Sidney Farber, quoted in "Magic Bullets," episode 1 of *Cancer: The Emperor of Maladies*, Public Broadcasting Service, 2015.

63 **Several of the new chemotherapy drugs . . .** American Cancer Society, "Evolution of Cancer Treatments: Chemotherapy," June 12, 2014, http://www.cancer.org/cancer/cancerbasics/thehistoryofcancer/the-history-of-cancer-cancer-treatment-chemo.

63 **"One could argue that . . ."** Jerome Yates, author's interview, August 12, 2014.

63 **As Emil Freireich pointed out . . .** "Magic Bullets," episode 1 of *Cancer: The Emperor of Maladies*, Public Broadcasting Service, 2015.

63 **"When the children were in remission, . . ."** "Children First: Dr. Donald Pinkel and the Quest to Cure Childhood Leukemia," *RPCI Alumni News,* Fall 2010–Winter 2011, https://www.roswellpark.org/sites/default/files/node-files/publication/nid91579-alumninews-winter10.pdf.

Chapter 11

66 **"The approach was to put in the time . . ."** Lucius Sinks, author's interview, May 22, 2015.

67 **"Or the bleeding would start . . ."** Emil Frei interview, NCI Oral History Project, June 3, 1997, 27–28, https://history.nih.gov/archives/downloads/freioralhistory.pdf.

67 **"Why don't you do something . . ."** Emil J. Freireich interview, NCI Oral History Project, June 19, 1997, 46, https://history.nih.gov/archives/downloads/freireich.pdf.

68 **At the time, the blood bank . . .** Frei interview, 28.

68 **"We may not cure leukemia . . ."** Frei interview, 29.

69 **"So what are we going to do . . ."** Freireich interview, 46.

69 **At first, patients were given . . .** Freireich interview, 66.

69 **"Oh, my God, . . ."** Freireich interview, 68.

70 **"All of us helped with it, . . ."** Frei interview, 32.

70 **Freireich said that Judson . . .** Freireich interview, 70. For a slide show of the early prototypes, see http://slidegur.com/doc/4972546/history-of-the-ibm-2990-2991-blood-separators.

70 **The hospital's new donor center, . . .** Sue Banchich, author's interview, October 18, 2015; Edwin A. Mirand, *Legacy and History of Roswell Park Cancer Institute, 1898–1998* (Virginia Beach: Donning Co., 1998), 83.

71 **"If anyone ever saw . . ."** Freireich interview, 63.

Chapter 12

73 **Susan, for example, remembered . . .** Susan Wendel Och, author's interview, August 12, 2014.

74 **"Are you making progress?"** Sinks, author's interview, May 22, 2015. All the quotations in this section of the chapter are from this interview.

Chapter 13

78 **In addition to being taken . . .** Alfred G. Gilman, Louis S. Goodman, Theodore W. Rall, and Ferid Murad, *The Pharmacological Basis of Therapeutics* (New York: Macmillan, 1985), 1246.

Chapter 14

83 **James Holland became a doctor . . .** James Holland, author's interview, January 29, 2015. All quotations from Holland in this chapter, unless otherwise noted, are from this interview.

83 **Early on at Delafield, . . .** John Laszlo, *The Cure of Childhood Leukemia: Into the Age of Miracles* (New Brunswick, NJ: Rutgers University Press, 1996), 214–15.

85 **Dr. Edwin Mirand, . . .** Edwin A. Mirand, *Legacy and History of Roswell Park Cancer Institute, 1898–1998* (Virginia Beach: Donning, 1998), 75.

86 **In the beginning, Pinkel said, . . .** Donald Pinkel, author's interview, October 22, 2013.

86 **"So we had to recruit patients . . ."** Emil J. Freireich interview, NCI Oral History Project, June 19, 1997, 44, https://history.nih.gov/archives/downloads/freireich.pdf.

87 **In 1965, he published . . .** James F. Holland, "Obstacles to the Control of Acute Leukemia," *CA: Cancer Journal for Clinicians* 15, no. 2 (1965): 85–89.

87 **"I need to talk to this man."** Jerome Yates, author's interview, August 12, 2014. All quotations from Yates in this chapter, unless otherwise noted, are from this interview.

89 **"A lot of it has to do with his voice, . . ."** Audrey Tuttolomondo, author's interview, October 10, 2014.

90 **Full many a gem . . .** "Elegy Written in a Country Churchyard," Thomas Gray, 1751. I was amazed that Holland could recite a verse, just off the top of his head, without much prompting. The entire poem can be found at http://www.poetryfoundation.org/poems-and-poets/poems/detail/44299.

91 **Dr. Larry Norton at Memorial Sloan Kettering . . .** Ronald Piana, "Managing Breast Cancer in 2015: A Conversation with Larry Norton," ASCOPost.com, May 25, 2015, http://www.ascopost.com/issues/may-25-2015/managing-breast-cancer-in-2015.aspx.

92 **"The clinical trials were key . . ."** Jerome Yates, author's interview, January 19, 2014.

93 **"This is because of the blood–brain . . ."** Donald Pinkel, author's interview, October 22, 2013.

Chapter 15

94 **When Donald Pinkel returned home . . .** Donald Pinkel, author's interview, August 22, 2014.

94 **After discussions about building . . .** Marlo Thomas interviewed by Larry King on "Larry King Live," December 9, 2005, archived at the Paley Center for Media, https://www.paleycenter.org/collection/item/?q=Marlo+Thomas&p=1&item=T:87770.

95 **"I boiled, boiled, boiled."** The story in this paragraph and following was found in Roswell Park Cancer Institute, "A Sense of Urgency: Donald Pinkel and the Quest to Cure ALL," accessed February 1, 2016, http://www.roswellpark.org/donaldpinkel.

97 **By the end of his first year, . . .** Marilyn Sadler, "Conquering Leukemia," *Memphis: The City Magazine*, February 1, 2012, http://memphismagazine.com/features/conquering-leukemia/.

97 **Despite early success, . . .** Hazel Fath, *A Dream Come True: The Story of St. Jude Children's Hospital and ALSAC* (Dallas: Taylor, 1983), 70; Donald Pinkel, author's interview, October 22, 2013.

Chapter 16

100 **"I brought you some homework."** Lucius Sinks, author's interview, February 20, 2015. All quotations in this chapter are from this interview.

100 **It was entitled *Conflicts in . . .*** Lucius F. Sinks and John O. Godden, *Conflicts in Childhood Cancer,* vol. 4 of *Progress in Clinical and Biological Research* (New York: A. R. Liss, 1975).

100 **And a tome it was.** James Holland and Emil Frei III, *Cancer Medicine,* 2nd ed. (New York: Lea & Febiger, 1982).

Chapter 17

104 **Eric's outpatient progress record** . . . Roswell Park Memorial Institute Out-Patient Records.
105 **"We knew the drugs were . . ."** Jane Wendel, author's interview, March 11, 2015.
108 **With that in mind, Holland began** . . . James Holland, author's interview, January 29, 2015; Jerome Yates, author's interview, August 12, 2014.
109 **"In the end, it doesn't matter, . . ."** Jerome Yates, author's interview, August 12, 2014.

Chapter 18

110 **Eight hundred feet at its deepest** . . . William Ratigan, *Great Lakes Shipwrecks and Survivals* (New York: Galahad Books, 1994), 283.
111 **"Dad just decided to go . . ."** Susan Wendel Och, author's interview, August 12, 2014.

Chapter 19

115 **After moving to Memphis** . . . Donald Pinkel, author's interview, August 22, 2014. All quotations in this chapter, unless otherwise noted, are from this interview.
115 **"Childhood lymphocytic leukemia . . ."** Donald Pinkel, Kathleen Hernandes, Luis Borella, Charlene Holton, Rhomes Aur, Gregory Savoy, and Charles Pratt, "Drug Dosage and Remission Duration in Childhood Lymphocytic Leukemia," *Cancer* 27, no. 2 (1971): 247–56, quotation on 255.
116 **"When you treat, you get rid of . . ."** Emil Frei interview, NCI Oral History Project, June 3, 1997, 21, https://history.nih.gov/archives/downloads/freioralhistory.pdf.
116 **"It had never been done before."** Donald Pinkel, interview by Sue Banchich, Roswell Park, June 17, 2010.
117 **"The development of effective therapy . . ."** Gaston K. Rivera, Donald Pinkel, Joseph V. Simone, Michael L. Hancock, and William M. Crist, "Treatment of Acute Lymphoblastic Leukemia: 30 Years' Experience at St. Jude Children's Research Hospital," *New England Journal of Medicine* 329 (1993): 1289–95.
117 **Decades later, James Holland told me** . . . James Holland, email interview with author and Jerry Yates, January 17, 2015.
117 **At St. Jude, radiation dosages** . . . Rivera et al., "Treatment of Acute Lymphoblastic Leukemia," 1290.
117 **In addition, 54 percent** . . . Thomas C. Pomeroy and Ralph E. Johnson, "Combined Modality Therapy of Acute Lymphocytic Leukemia," *Cancer* 35, no. 1 (1975): 36–47.

117 **Holland's group in Buffalo** . . . James Holland, author's interview, January 29, 2015.
117 **"The cost of the cure, . . ."** Lucius Sinks, author's interview, May 22, 2015.

Chapter 20

118 **"How old were you . . ."** Donald Pinkel, phone conversation with the author, June 14, 2015. All quotations in this chapter, unless otherwise noted, are from this conversation.
119 **"It was not unusual to hit rough weather . . ."** Susan Wendel Och, author's interview, August 12, 2014.

Chapter 21

122 **"It reminds me too much of my brother."** Being a parent makes one vulnerable in new and sometimes painful ways. It took me a long time to wrap my mind around that concept. When my son, Chris, was sick as a child, it transported me back to the leukemia years with Eric.

Chapter 22

127 **The formidable ridge of land** . . . Pierre Berton, *Niagara: A History of the Falls* (New York: Penguin Books), 12–15. Growing up, I sometimes watched Berton on Canadian television. He was a respected social commentator in that country and wrote nearly forty books. Our house on Canal Road was 20 miles from Niagara Falls, and we visited several times during my childhood. Berton's book helped me understand the history and majesty in my own backyard.
132 **"That's what I call teamwork, . . ."** That game against the Depew Saints soon became the stuff of legend in our household. I remember being there with my father, but my brother Chris also remembered being there, and the story was told and retold so many times it soon seemed like the whole family was there that day.
134 **By Eric's second season** . . . Jane Wendel, author's interview, March 11, 2015.

Chapter 23

136 **The headline would be** . . . Roland H. Berg, "We Have a Chance to Beat Leukemia Now," *Look*, May 5, 1970, 26–31. In teaching my classes at Johns Hopkins

University, I came across an interview with Laura Hillenbrand about how she used old newspapers and magazines when writing her books *Unbroken* and *Seabiscuit*. Hillenbrand suffers from chronic fatigue syndrome, or CFS, and rarely travels, so the publications from the past become like a time machine. She gleans as much from the adjoining stories and advertisements as she does the specific articles themselves. For this major day in Roswell Park history, I purchased a copy of *Look* magazine on eBay for $3.50. It was money well spent because that era again came alive for me as I flipped through the pages.

136 **"That *Look* article was . . ."** Lucius Sinks, author's interview, February 20, 2015.

137 **"A fatal disease shows signs . . ."** Berg, "We Have a Chance to Beat Leukemia Now," 27.

138 **"We ended up meeting . . ."** Jimmie Holland, author's interview, January 29, 2015. All quotations in this chapter, unless otherwise noted, are from this interview.

139 **"They have measured everything . . ."** In Jimmie Holland and Sheldon Lewis, *The Human Side of Cancer: Living with Hope, Coping with Uncertainty* (New York: HarperCollins, 2000), 7.

140 **She defines "palliative care" . . .** Ibid., 253.

140 **According to the National Cancer Institute . . .** National Cancer Institute, "Palliative Care in Cancer," 2010, https://www.cancer.gov/about-cancer/advanced-cancer/care-choices/palliative-care-fact-sheet.

140 **"When it comes to cancer care . . ."** Suzanne Gordon, conversation with the author, August 5, 2016.

141 **Dr. Martin Brecher recalled . . .** Martin Brecher, author's interview, October 20, 2015.

141 **Here, framed photographs of celebrities . . .** Edwin A. Mirand, *Legacy and History of Roswell Park Cancer Institute, 1898–1998* (Virginia Beach: Donning, 1998), 82.

Chapter 24

148 **A full-page advertisement . . .** In Siddhartha Mukherjee, *The Emperor of All Maladies: A Biography of Cancer* (New York: Scribner, 2010), 180.

148 **Mary Lasker, a lobbyist, . . .** Ibid., 185–86.

149 **"Your brother was at Roswell Park . . ."** Lucius Sinks, author's interview, May 22, 2015. All quotations in this chapter, unless otherwise noted, are from this interview.

151 **Martell's father, . . .** "One Death Inspires $15 Million Cancer Fight," *New York Times*, June 8, 1986.

152 **In January 1972, Kevin Garvey . . .** Kevin Guest House, "Kevin's Story," 2017, http://www.kevinguesthouse.org/ourstory.asp.

Chapter 25

155 **"I had been head nurse . . ."** Audrey Tuttolomondo, author's interview, October 10, 2014.

156 **It helped to have a sense of humor . . .** Jerome Yates, author's interview, August 12, 2014.

156 **Keep them safe from infection . . .** Vince DeVita, *Fresh Air with Terry Gross*, National Public Radio, October 28, 2015, http://www.npr.org/2015/10/28/452395967/oncologist-discusses-advancements-in-treatment-and-the-ongoing-war-on-cancer. See also Vince DeVita and Elizabeth DeVita-Raeburn, *The Death of Cancer: After Fifty Years on the Front Lines of Medicine, a Pioneering Oncologist Reveals Why the War on Cancer Is Winnable—and How We Can Get There* (New York: Farrar, Straus, and Giroux, 2015), 163.

156 **"[Children] are extremely resilient . . ."** Jerome Yates, author's interview, August 12, 2014.

156 **Also, Jimmie Holland soon noticed . . .** Jimmie Holland, author's interview, January 29, 2015.

157 **In looking at the responses . . .** Jimmie Holland, Marjorie Plumb, Jerome Yates, Sandra Harris, Audrey Tuttolomondo, Josephine Holmes, and James F. Holland, "Psychological Response of Patients with Acute Leukemia to Germ-Free Environments," *Cancer* 40, no. 2 (1977): 871–79.

157 **In a subsequent report, Yates stated that . . .** In Lucius F. Sinks and John O. Godden, *Conflicts in Childhood Cancer*, vol. 4 of *Progress in Clinical and Biological Research* (New York: A. R. Liss, 1975), 322.

Chapter 26

158 **On this summer afternoon, . . .** Susan Wendel Och, author's interview, August 12, 2014, and Chris Wendel, author's interview, November 14, 2014. All quotations in this chapter, unless otherwise noted, are from these interviews.

160 **A physical examination "revealed . . ."** Roswell Park Memorial Institute Out-Patient Records.

161 **"Dogs are our link to paradise. . . ."** Attributed to Milan Kundera, https://www.goodreads.com/quotes/37510-dogs-are-our-link-to-paradise-they-don-t-know-evil. This is likely a pastiche of thoughts and words from Tereza's musings on her dog, Karenin, in Kundera, *The Unbearable Lightness of Being* (New York: Harper and Row, 1984).

Chapter 27

165 **On October 11, 1971, . . .** Hearings at Roswell Park, National Cancer Attack Act of 1971: Hearings, Ninety-Second Congress, First Session, on H.R. 8343,

H.R. 10681, S. 1828. All the quotations in this chapter, unless otherwise noted, are from this source.

166 **As the *Chicago Tribune* noted, . . .** "Tower Ticker," *Chicago Tribune*, January 28, 1971.

167 **Sitting behind a small wooden desk, . . .** The American Presidency Project, "Richard Nixon: Remarks on Signing the National Cancer Act of 1971, December 23, 1971," accessed July 21, 2017, http://www.presidency.ucsb.edu/ws/?pid=3275.

168 **With a stroke of the presidential pen, . . .** Lucius Sinks, author's interview, May 22, 2015.

Chapter 28

169 **As Tom Junod wrote in *Esquire* . . .** Tom Junod, "The Death of Patient Zero," *Esquire*, August 2015, 108. This was part of an amazing series of stories about the role of medicine in modern life.

170 **"Every time I took Eric . . ."** Jane Wendel, author's interview, March 11, 2015.

170 **"When you're putting a patient, . . ."** Cheryl Tabone, author's interview, July 14, 2015.

171 **Instead of high doses . . .** Arnold I. Freeman et al., "Comparison of Intermediate-Dose Methotrexate with Cranial Irradiation for Post-Induction Treatment of Acute Lymphocytic Leukemia in Children," *New England Journal of Medicine* 308 (1983).

171 **Instead an "intermediate dose" . . .** Lucius F. Sinks, Jaw J. Wang, and Arnold Freeman, "The Treatment of Primary Childhood Acute Lymphocytic Leukemia with Intermediate Dose Methotrexate," *Haematology and Blood Transfusion* 26 (1981): 99–107.

172 **The toxicity of the intermediate dose . . .** Freeman et al., "Comparison of Intermediate-Dose Methotrexate with Cranial Irradiation."

Chapter 29

174 **Old-timers down at the Olcott Yacht Club . . .** William Ratigan, *Great Lakes Shipwrecks and Survivals* (New York: Galahad Books, 1994), 293–94.

174 **"It occurred just as the sun . . ."** Ibid., 301–2.

Chapter 30

179 **After graduating from Niagara University . . .** Catherine Lyons, author's interview, November 2, 2015.

180 **"Our nurses were right there . . ."** James Holland, author's interview, November 19, 2014.

180 **Brenda Hall went to Sweet Home . . .** Brenda Hall, author's interview, December 12, 2014.

180 **One father, a dapper-dressed . . .** Jane Wendel, author's interview, March 11, 2015.

181 **"We must be doing right . . ."** Ibid.

181 **"She got their minds . . ."** Brenda Hall, author's interview, December 12, 2014.

Chapter 31

182 **The National Hockey League . . .** Hockey Reference, "1972 NHL Amateur Draft," accessed July 17, 2017, http://www.hockey-reference.com/draft/ NHL_1972_amateur.html. For Jim Schoenfeld's bio, see Hockey Reference, "Jim Schoenfeld," accessed July 17, 2017, http://www.hockey-reference.com/players/s/ schoeji01.html.

183 **"We had decided that we . . ."** Jane Wendel, author's interview, March 11, 2015. All quotations in this chapter, unless otherwise noted, are from this interview.

183 **"Today we know so much more . . ."** Donald Pinkel, phone interview with author, August 1, 2015.

184 **It was a study . . .** Donald Pinkel, "Chickenpox and Leukemia," *Journal of Pediatrics* 58 (1961): 729–37.

184 **On December 5, 1972, . . .** Eric Wendel patient summary.

185 **The Boston Bruins, . . .** Joe Pelletier, "Jim Schoenfeld," Greatest Hockey Legends.com, accessed July 17, 2007, http://sabreslegends.blogspot.com/2007/06/ jim-schoenfeld.html. A YouTube video of the fight with Wayne Cashman can be found at https://www.youtube.com/watch?v=e1zbVjjOG7o.

187 **But in recent years, David Bowie, . . .** Ian Shapira, "What Kind of Cancer Killed Them? Obituaries for David Bowie and Others Don't Say," *Washington Post*, January 22, 2016.

Chapter 32

189 **Eric was discharged . . .** Jane Wendel, author's interview, March 11, 2015. All quotations in this chapter, unless otherwise noted, are from this interview.

189 **To reach the Purple Room . . .** Peter Wendel, author's interview, October 30, 2015.

192 **On March 1, 1973, . . .** Eric Wendel patient summary.

192 **"We took off our shoes, . . ."** Susan Wendel Och, author's interview, August 12, 2014.
193 **"I remember," he said** . . . Jim Schoenfeld, author's interview, April 2, 2012.

Chapter 33

195 **All I know is** . . . "Jim Harrison: By the Book," *New York Times*, Book Review, March 17, 2016.

Chapter 35

199 **"That right?"** . . . Lucius Sinks, author's interview, May 22, 2015.

Chapter 36

203 **"Soon after your brother, . . ."** Lucius Sinks, author's interview, September 25, 2015.
203 **As Holland remembered it** . . . James Holland, author's interview, November 19, 2015.
205 **Fifteen department heads** . . . Barbara J. Culliton, "Academics in New York and California Fight Disclosure Policies," *Science* 196, no. 4285 (1977): 37–38.
205 **None of the doctors** . . . In "Noted Researcher Leaving Roswell, Hits State Attitude," *Courier-Express*, June 30, 1976.
205 **The *Courier-Express*, . . .** "State Doctors Should Bare Finances," *Courier-Express*, July 2, 1976.
205 **The *Buffalo Evening News* . . .** "Morale Problem for Roswell," *Buffalo Evening News*, July 1, 1976.
206 **"I don't have any problems . . ."** In Barbara J. Culliton, "Academics in New York and California Fight Disclosure Policies," *Science* 196, no. 4285 (1977): 37.
206 **"The plaintiffs are employed . . ."** Evans v. Carey, 53 A.D.2d 109 1976, https://scholar.google.com/scholar_case?case=16019974660532786838&hl=en&as_sdt=6&as_vis=1&oi=scholarr.
206 **"True, and many others . . ."** Lucius Sinks, author's interview, September 25, 2015.
207 **Study No. 7611, . . .** Arnold I. Freeman et al., "Comparison of Intermediate-Dose Methotrexate with Cranial Irradiation for Post-Induction Treatment of Acute Lymphocytic Leukemia in Children," *New England Journal of Medicine* 308 (1983).
208 **In the last line of the article** . . . Ibid.

208 **In a 1997 follow-up study, . . .** Arnold I. Freeman, James M. Boyett, Arvin S. Glicksman, Martin L. Brecher, Brigit G. Leventhal, Lucius F. Sinks, and James F. Holland, "Intermediate-Dose Methotrexate versus Cranial Irradiation in Childhood Acute Lymphoblastic Leukemia: A Ten-Year Follow-Up," *Medical and Pediatric Oncology* 28, no. 2 (1997), http://dx.doi.org/10.1002/(SICI)1096-911X(199702)28:2<98::AID-MPO3>3.0.CO;2-N.

208 **Gregory Armstrong . . .** In *ASCO Daily News*, "Changes in Pediatric Cancer Treatments Yield Reduced Late Mortality," May 31, 2015, https://am.asco.org/changes-pediatric-cancer-treatments-yield-reduced-late-mortality.

209 **Michael Link . . .** Ibid.

209 **"Given the increasing . . ."** Arnold I. Freeman et al., "Comparison of Intermediate-Dose Methotrexate with Cranial Irradiation for Post-Induction Treatment of Acute Lymphocytic Leukemia in Children," *New England Journal of Medicine* 308 (1983).

209 **So it was . . .** Arnold I. Freeman, James M. Boyett, Arvin S. Glicksman, Martin L. Brecher, Brigit G. Leventhal, Lucius F. Sinks, and James F. Holland, "Intermediate-Dose Methotrexate versus Cranial Irradiation in Childhood Acute Lymphoblastic Leukemia: A Ten-Year Follow-Up," *Medical and Pediatric Oncology* 28, no. 2 (1997).

210 **After realizing that . . .** Eugene W. Straus and Alex Straus, *Medical Marvels: The 100 Greatest Advances in Medicine* (Amherst, NY: Prometheus Books, 2006), 269.

Chapter 38

215 **My brother Bryan . . .** Bryan Wendel, author's interview, February 1, 2016.

215 **Chris said he thinks . . .** Chris Wendel, author's interview, November 14, 2014.

216 **"When asked what . . ."** Amy Foster, email interview, June 24, 2017.

216 **"In the latitude to . . ."** Susan Wendel Och, author's interview, August 12, 2014.

Further Readings

Bailey, Budd. *Today in Buffalo Sports History: 366 Days of Milestones.* Buffalo: Buffalo Books, 2013.

Barnes, Julian. *Levels of Life.* New York: Alfred A. Knopf, 2013.

Berton, Pierre. *Niagara: A History of the Falls.* New York: Penguin Books, 1992.

Davis, Wade. *Into the Silence: The Great War, Mallory, and the Conquest of Everest.* New York: Vintage, 2012.

Deford, Frank. *Alex: The Life of a Child.* New York: New American Library and Viking Press, 1997.

DeVita, Vincent T., Jr., and Elizabeth DeVita-Raeburn. *The Death of Cancer: After Fifty Years on the Front Lines of Medicine, a Pioneering Oncologist Reveals Why the War on Cancer Is Winnable—and How We Can Get There.* New York: Farrar, Straus and Giroux, 2015.

Didion, Joan. *Blue Nights.* London: Fourth Estate, 2011.

Fath, Hazel. *A Dream Come True: The Story of St. Jude Children's Research Hospital and ALSAC.* Dallas: Taylor, 1983.

Freireich, Emil J., and Noreen A. Lemak. *Milestones in Leukemia Research and Therapy.* Baltimore: Johns Hopkins University Press, 1991.

Gilman, Alfred Goodman, Louis S. Goodman, Theodore W. Rall, and Ferid Murad. *The Pharmacological Basis of Therapeutics.* 7th ed. New York: Macmillan, 1985.

Gladwell, Malcolm. *David and Goliath: Underdogs, Misfits and the Art of Battling Giants.* New York: Little Brown, 2013.

Hanh, Thich Nhat. *Old Path White Clouds: Walking in the Footsteps of the Buddha.* Berkeley: Parallax Press, 1991.

Holland, James, and Emil Frei III. *Cancer Medicine.* 2nd ed. New York: Lea & Febiger, 1982.

Holland, Jimmie, and Sheldon Lewis. *The Human Side of Cancer: Living with Hope, Coping with Uncertainty*. New York: HarperCollins, 2000.

Kalanithi, Paul. *When Breath Becomes Air*. New York: Random House, 2016.

Laszlo, John. *The Cure of Childhood Leukemia: Into the Age of Miracles*. New Brunswick, NJ: Rutgers University Press, 1996.

Maclean, Norman. *A River Runs through It and Other Stories*. Chicago: University of Chicago Press, 1976.

Mirand, Edwin. *Legacy and History of Roswell Park Cancer Institute, 1898–1998*. Virginia Beach: Donning Co., 1998.

Mukherjee, Siddhartha. *The Emperor of All Maladies: A Biography of Cancer*. New York: Scribner, 2010.

Oates, Joyce Carol. *The Lost Landscape: A Writer's Coming of Age*. New York: Ecco, 2015.

Ratigan, William. *Great Lakes Shipwrecks and Survivals*. New York: Galahad Books, 1994.

Sinks, Lucius, and John O. Godden. *Conflicts in Childhood Cancer*. Vol. 4 of *Progress in Clinical and Biological Research*. New York: Alan R. Liss, 1975.

Sissman, L. E. *Hello, Darkness: The Collected Poems of L. E. Sissman*. Boston: Atlantic Monthly Press, 1963.

Skloot, Rebecca. *The Immortal Life of Henrietta Lacks*. New York: Broadway Books, 2010.

Stockton, Robert. *Roswell Park: A Memoir*. Ithaca, NY: Cornell University Library Digital Collections, 2008.

Straus, Eugene W., and Alex Straus. *Medical Marvels: The 100 Greatest Advances in Medicine*. Amherst, NY: Prometheus Books, 2006.

Vowell, Sarah. *Assassination Vacation*. New York: Simon & Schuster, 2005.

Tim Wendel is the award-winning author of thirteen books, including *Summer of '68, Castro's Curveball,* and *High Heat,* which was an Editor's Choice selection by the *New York Times Book Review.* A writer-in-residence at Johns Hopkins University, his stories have appeared in the *New York Times,* the *Washington Post, National Geographic, Washingtonian, Gargoyle, GQ,* and *Esquire.* www.timwendel.com